Patsy Westcott is one
· magazine's top j

By the same author

Pregnancy and Birth
Your Child's Health
Feeding Your Baby and Child

The
Mother & Baby
Book of

YOUR BABY'S
FIRST YEAR

Patsy Westcott

GRAFTON BOOKS
A Division of the Collins Publishing Group

LONDON GLASGOW
TORONTO SYDNEY AUCKLAND

Grafton Books
A Division of the Collins Publishing Group
8 Grafton Street, London W1X 3LA

A Grafton Paperback Original 1990

A catalogue record for this
book is available from the British Library

ISBN 0-586-20662-0

Printed and bound in Great Britain by
Collins, Glasgow

Set in Goudy Old Style

CONTENTS

INTRODUCTION

I well remember coming home from hospital with my first baby. There was a sense of exhilaration and pride that 'I'd done it'. However, after the congratulations and excitement of the birth had died down I was assailed by a sense of panic – if only my baby had been issued with a book of instructions! It was around that time that I picked up my first copy of *Mother & Baby* magazine. Then, as now, it was packed with advice and information for every parent – the sense of relief was enormous.

Today, as one of M&B's regular contributors I'm well aware that there are still new mothers out there longing for that instruction book. I hope that this book will go some way to meeting that need. It guides you through those first weeks at home, weeks of joy and confusion. It contains helpful tips on how to care for your baby and yet still make time for yourself – vital for every new mother. Newborn babies spend a lot of their time feeding, so there is a section in this book devoted to breast- and bottle-feeding, including some of the problems you might encounter and how to solve them.

Part three looks at two more subjects that preoccupy new parents – sleeping and crying. Most parents worry that their babies don't do enough of the first, and do too much of the second! This section helps you know when to worry and suggests how gently to guide your baby into a more civilized sleeping pattern. It also gives plenty of tried and tested hints for soothing him when he cries.

One of the most rewarding parts of being a parent is watching your baby grow and develop. Your child will never again change so quickly as in the first year when every day brings some new skill or ability. Part four tells you what to expect so that you can get the most out of your baby's development and be reassured that it is normal. Finally we look at some of the minor ailments that might occur during your baby's first year, and offer advice on how you can keep your baby healthy.

If this book helps you to have a relaxed and enjoyable first year, it will have succeeded in its purpose.

Happy first year! Patsy Westcott, 1990

Note: In order to reflect the experiences of all mothers, 'he' and 'she' have been alternated chapter by chapter in this book to refer to the baby.

Part I

GETTING TO KNOW YOU

First weeks at home

The birth of a first baby marks a turning point in your life. From now on you are a parent, you have a family, and everything you do, say or think will be influenced by this new situation.

The first weeks at home with your new baby are a time of adjustment. You and your husband have to become used to having another member of the family and to the idea that you are now totally responsible for another human being. During these settling-in weeks you may feel completely exhausted. This isn't caused only by the hard physical work that goes into looking after a baby, but by the mental strain involved in such a major change in your life. As you become more used to being a mother, as the everyday tasks of baby care come more easily to you and your baby becomes more settled, you will find you regain your energy.

Looking after your baby
At first, the basic jobs of simply caring for your baby – feeding, changing and keeping him clean – will take up most of your time. You will find advice on how to cope in the chapters that follow. Don't expect too much of yourself at the beginning. After all, if you had just started a new job, you wouldn't expect to be able to cope with every aspect of it right away. It's the same with motherhood.

As a mother you are cook, cleaner, laundry maid, nurse, chauffeur, teacher, companion and playmate. Yet, as a job, motherhood has very little recognition afforded to it. You are not paid, and the rest of the world seems to be unaware of the difficulties of getting around with a pram or pushchair or of snatching a few precious hours to yourself. You may miss the company of your workmates; yet the latest office gossip seems less important to you now than knowing how to deal with broken nights or three-month colic (see page 60). In short, your life has undergone a revolution. It is hardly surprising if at times you feel bewildered and wonder whether you have done the right thing.

At the same time, being a parent brings enormous, often intangible rewards. The sight of your baby's first gummy smile, watching him grow and develop and knowing that you have contributed to the progress of this little human being, can give you a deeply satisfying sense of achievement.

The secret of coping in the early months is to achieve a balance between sorting out the practical aspects of baby care and making space for yourself and the other members of your family.

Making friends
Other mothers can be an enormous source of practical support and friendship when you have a baby and young children. Some of the friends you make now could well last a lifetime as you share each other's joys and sorrows.

Ask your health visitor whether there are any postnatal groups in your area, such as those run by the National Childbirth Trust or Meet-a-Mum Association (addresses on page 139). Now that you no longer go out to work, you will probably discover neighbours you never knew existed, some of whom will also have small children. There may be a babysitting circle in your area, which is a good source of friends as well as giving you the opportunity for a much-needed break. Again, your health visitor should know of such groups in your area, or look on the clinic noticeboard or in your local library, health centre or community centre.

Check out your local toddler group too. Despite its name, babies are just as welcome, and you will meet many other mothers in the same situation as yourself.

Establishing a routine
A newborn baby is naturally unsettled. One day he sleeps calmly between feeds, the next he seems to do nothing but cry. Sometimes you are at your wits' end to know what to do with him. At times like this it helps to have people to call on who understand what you are talking about. Your health visitor, too, is a useful ally.

Even though your baby is unpredictable try to get out of the house at least once a day. If you are breast-feeding you don't need to worry if he wakes up for a feed, as you can simply put him to the breast wherever you are. Most people won't even notice you are feeding. If you are bottle-feeding you will need to be a little more organized when you go out. Put a couple of bottles of made-up feed from the fridge into an insulated bag, together with a flask of hot water and a bowl to warm up the feeds, and you're ready to go.

Gradually over the course of the next few weeks your baby will become more regular in his habits. You will know, more or less, when you can expect him to wake for a feed, play, and so on; and as this happens your routine will become easier to plan. By the time your baby is three months old most of the worrying inconsistencies in his behaviour will have disappeared, and you will both be more used to each other.

How to cope in the early weeks

- Rule number one for new parents: learn to tolerate dust! If you can relax your housework standards until your baby is more settled, you will make life easier for yourself than if you worry about every speck of dirt.
- Follow your baby's lead. You will cope much more easily if you comply with your baby's wants and needs at this early age. You cannot spoil a new baby because he is unable to distinguish between his wants and needs. If you feed him when he wants feeding, comfort him when he can't sleep and generally devote yourself to him, you will find he settles down more easily and quickly.
- Get out of the house as often as you can. Once your baby is more settled you can have a flexible schedule; for instance, clinic one afternoon, visit to friends the next, toddler group the next, visitors to you, and so on. Variety is the spice of life when you have a baby.
- If you feel under pressure and unable to cope, talk about it with your health visitor.

NOW YOU ARE A FAMILY

Your other children

If you have other children you may find you cope more easily with your new baby this time around. You have the advantage of experience, and your baby picks up your relaxed attitude and settles more quickly into family life.

Your other children's reactions to the new baby will depend on their ages, stages of development and individual personalities. It is a rare family that doesn't experience some sibling rivalry (the term used by experts for conflict between brothers and sisters) during the baby years or later on in childhood.

If your children are close together you will have two lots of nappies and two lots of broken nights to cope with. On the other hand, many parents prefer to deal with the baby stage during a short period rather than to stretch it out over the course of years. A child under the age of three is unable to make his jealousy easily known. So he may appear loving and affectionate towards the baby and then, when your back is turned, aim a punch at him or kiss him overenthusiastically. In these cases, although you will find it difficult, you should respond to the feeling behind the action rather than the bad behaviour itself. Of course, you should not allow your toddler to hurt the new baby, but you should also show him that you love him, and reassure him that your affection for him hasn't waned.

Your husband can play an important part in making your toddler feel wanted and involved. He can take him out for special trips on his own, or play games with him that cannot include the baby. You, too, can help reassure him by involving him in the care of the baby – many young toddlers show a real desire to help and often become surprisingly skilful at interpreting the baby's needs and wants. Try to make a special time each day when you can be alone with your toddler; and cope calmly if he reverts to earlier habits such as wetting his pants even though he was previously potty trained.

With careful handling your baby and your toddler will form a firm friendship that will probably last a lifetime.

You and your partner

The relationship with your husband is bound to change in the early years. In some ways the marriage has to go on automatic pilot while you work out your new relationships; for though children are a source of enormous joy and rewards, they can also be a strain at times.

Perhaps for the first time in your married life you and your husband inhabit separate worlds. He is out at work all day, while your life revolves round babies and children. What's more, if you are not planning to go back to work your husband may feel the strain of being the sole breadwinner. He may wonder whether he will be able to cope, or he may feel trapped into being a family man when he doesn't feel ready for it. It's not that he doesn't want to be a father, simply that, like you, he may feel he's reached the point of no return. Bear with these feelings and talk to each other; most couples go through them, and in sharing the good times as well as the bad you may even strengthen the bond between you.

Sometimes the arrival of a baby can spark off more deep-seated insecurities, perhaps associated with the time when a brother or sister

---

Happy families – coping with a new baby when you have other children

- Stay in hospital for as short a time as possible.
- Don't move the baby into the cot that has just been left by the toddler for he is bound to feel usurped. Make any moves from cot to big bed well in advance of the baby's arrival.
- Keep a store of little presents and give them to your toddler when visitors arrive bearing gifts for the baby, so he won't feel left out.
- Try to keep to your toddler's usual routine.
- Make sure you spend some time alone with your other children when the baby is not around.
- Let older children help you care for the baby.
- A little forethought makes for happier feed times – while you are feeding the baby make sure your toddler's potty and a drink are on hand, and that you have a book you can look at together or a special toy for him to play with.
- Intercede between your toddler and visitors if they pay all their attention to the baby and none to him.
- If there is a small age gap between your baby and toddler, the early months will be difficult. Remember it does get better.

---

was born. Your husband may be jealous of your bond with the baby and wonder where he fits in. There is no magic formula to pull you through these transitions, but keeping the lines of communication open and learning how to handle disagreements constructively will help.

If you feel out of your depth, or the problems become too difficult to handle, you may benefit from professional help and advice from your doctor or a marriage guidance counsellor.

The new father

During the course of recent years the role of the father has changed, and he has become much more involved in the day-to-day process of child care. However, although most fathers are now present at the birth and play a more active part once their wives come home from hospital, women still do the lion's share of the work of looking after the baby. The situation must sometimes appear to be very confusing for the modern father. He doesn't know what is really expected of him.

So what should you do if you're a father with a new baby? There are no rules, so it is up to you and your wife to work out between you the level of involvement that is practical and suits both of you. For example, where earning a living comes into conflict with giving the night feeds, most men opt out. It is not surprising. It is arguably easier for a mother at home to catch up on her sleep during the day than for the father at the office. But then a vicious circle forms: the mother becomes ever more expert at the child-care tasks and father takes more and more of a back seat.

If you find this is happening in your household and it is making you unhappy, you will need to talk about it and work out practical ways of sharing the jobs more equally between you. For instance, perhaps father could give the night feeds at the weekend.

In practice each couple tends to work out their own compromise. Perhaps the baby's father always gives him his bath or tucks him up in bed, while his mother prepares the evening meal. Alternatively, the father may babysit for a couple of evenings while the mother has a breather.

Apart from breast-feeding there is nothing a mother can do for a baby that a father cannot do just as well, given the practice and the opportunity. Bear in mind that if you want equal involvement you will have to be prepared to accept that you will each do things differently. It can help to have previously discussed your respective ideas about

---

Survival tips for new parents

- Spend some time together every day, even if it's only a few minutes sitting over a cup of tea when the children have gone to bed.
- Sort out any money worries. Discuss whether you would be better off with a joint bank account or separate accounts, and work out painless ways of paying bills. Money can become all too easily a bone of contention between married couples, if you let it.
- Talk to each other about your hopes and feelings about child rearing, and try to trace the origins of your ideas. People often carry on the patterns they picked up in their own families without examining them. If your ideas differ vastly they can be a source of conflict.
- Learn how to manage disagreements. When your plans and needs conflict you will need to negotiate. Perhaps you could take it in turns to babysit, allowing one of you to engage in some other activity. Alternatively, you may need to come to a compromise – your husband spends only two hours playing cricket while you look after the baby and in return he babysits while you go to a keep-fit class. The important thing is not to let disagreements fester; defuse tension before it has time to build up.
- Make time for each other. Try to get out together without the baby at least once a week. You may not find it easy but it will do you the world of good, and the effort is really worth while.

bringing up children. A flexible, tolerant attitude is the secret of success.

You may decide that you would like to keep to strictly separate spheres, with the mother taking responsibility for home and family and the father for earning a living. In reality the roles tend to become blurred, even in households where couples accept the traditional arrangement. Father often spends time playing with the baby, for example. In fact, fathers who have made the effort to be close to their children often speak of the special joy and satisfaction they derive from their relationships.

Tips for new fathers

- Don't be put off by other people's remarks. Sometimes members of an older generation may be discouraging about your efforts to be involved in looking after your baby. Don't allow them to bother you – times have changed.
- Make the most of your time with the baby – it's quality not quantity that counts. Watch him to see what games you could play together, and what things he likes best.
- Don't be afraid to show your baby affection. He will love it when you cuddle him and give him interesting things to look at.
- You can be responsible for all sorts of jobs – changing the baby's nappy, giving him a bath, rocking him in your arms, taking him in the pram for a walk.
- Child-care experts agree that a baby can share just as strong a bond with his father as with his mother – given the opportunity.

Sleeping

If your budget will run to it a basic crib or Moses basket is useful for the first few weeks of your baby's life. It will fit in easily next to your bed so you can lift your baby out of it for night feeds, and it can be used elsewhere in the house. An alternative, if you can't afford a crib or basket, is to use the top of his carrycot or pram. From the age of about four to six months your baby will need a proper cot. There are many varieties available. The sort that has a movable mattress base is useful, to minimize wear and tear on your back! A drop-side is convenient too. Consider also buying the type of cot that later converts into a bed. Once your baby is big enough you can remove the cot sides without the disruption of putting her in a 'big bed'.

EQUIPMENT GUIDE

Babies seem to need an alarming amount of equipment. It's not easy
when you're a novice parent to decide what is essential. Over the next
few pages are listed some of the items you might find useful. But, as in
everything else, be guided by your baby's needs.

General equipment

- Carrycot, crib, Moses basket and/or cot
- Waterproof mattress covering for crib and/or cot
- Two or three fitted sheets for mattress
- Duvet or cellular blankets
- Carrying shawl or baby nest
- Cot and/or crib lining to make your baby feel secure and prevent her hurting her head if she bumps it on the cot/crib sides
- Pram or carrycot with wheels
- Pushchair
- Sling and/or baby carrier for when she is bigger
- Baby bath and stand, or large washing-up bowl
- Large towel with or without hood
- Changing mat
- Toiletries
- Nappies (disposable or fabric)
- Nappy liners
- Safety pins
- Plastic pants
- Two covered nappy buckets
- Baby seat
- Highchair
- Weaning spoons
- Plastic bowls
- Different types of bib

For breast-feeding

- 3 adjustable nursing bras, preferably made of cotton or cotton mix
- Thick breast pads (not plastic backed)
- Couple of bottles with teats (for drinks of water or juice)
- Sterilizing tablets or fluid
- Breast pump (optional) for expressing breast milk to leave if you go out without your baby
- Packet of baby milk (if you prefer to leave formula when you go out)

For bottle-feeding

- 6 large (300 ml or 8–9 fl. oz.) bottles, with caps and teats
- Measuring jug
- Bottle brush
- Sterilizing kit
- Sterilizing solution or tablets

Out and about

The sort of pram you choose depends on your pocket and your lifestyle, as well as the number of children you plan to have. A coach-built carriage pram is comfortable for the baby, easy for you to push around and durable enough to use for several babies. However, if you live in a small flat up several flights of stairs, it's obviously impractical as it takes up a lot of storage space and you may find it difficult to manoeuvre.

If you want something that is easy to store and that folds up so you can put it in the back of a car, the type of pram that looks like a carrycot on wheels is ideal. The degrees of comfort and sophistication available vary depending on how much you are prepared to pay.

Pushchairs – safety tips

- Check the label to ensure that it conforms to British Standard safety requirements – by law pushchairs must conform to BS 4792.
- Don't ever hang shopping bags from the handle.
- Always check the brakes are firmly on before leaving a pushchair.
- Take care when opening and closing the pushchair or adjusting the seat as fingers can easily get trapped.

To lull her to sleep

- Hammock-style baby rocker
- Pram rocker
- Lambskin
- Soother tape

Another practical option is the three-in-one type of pram, which is basically a carrycot on wheels that converts to a pushchair. Its only disadvantages are that it is not so comfy for your baby and may not be durable enough to use for more than a couple of children.

When choosing a pushchair, check it for ease of folding and storing, especially if you are likely to be using it on public transport. If you have no car, you will need a pushchair that has plenty of space for shopping. Swivel wheels are easier to manage than the straight variety, but check that they can lock into a straight position.

A simple, basic pushchair consists of straight wheels, no shopping tray and no option to recline it for when your baby is young, or sleeping. That means you can't really use it before your baby is six months old.

Next in the line are lie-back pushchairs which have an adjustable back to enable your baby to recline if she falls asleep. The fully reclining type of pushchair can be used instead of a pram, although it may not be practical in winter as it does not afford much protection for your baby.

Car safety

- Rearward-facing plastic shell – can be used for newborn baby on front or back seat
- Carrycot with straps
- Recliner seat to be used with back seat belts
- Car seat with fixings
- Car seat with handle – also converts to rocking seat

Other aids and equipment

- Simple bouncing chair
- Bouncer/rocking chair
- Baby bouncer that clamps or screws to doorframe
- Circular walking frame
- Inflatable baby walker
- Wooden slatted playpen with built-in base
- Panelled playpen
  Avoid lobster-pot playpens with V-shaped support legs as there have been fatal accidents involved with using them.

CARING FOR YOUR NEW BABY

BATHTIME

You will have been shown how to bath your baby if you attended antenatal classes and were probably given a 'refresher' demonstration before you left hospital.

New babies don't get very dirty, so there is no need to bath them every day. Many newborns feel insecure when undressed and dislike being bathed. If this applies to your baby you need only top and tail him (see page 15) until he grows more active and confident. Later on, in the first year, bathtime will become a time for fun and play together before bedtime.

STEP BY STEP TO BATHING YOUR BABY

1. Collect everything you need (see box) in the room in which you plan to bath your baby. If you have a radiator or heated towel rail put the clothes and towel over them to warm.

2. Fill the bath with 8–10 cm (3–4 in.) of warm water. Always put cold water in first and top up with hot. The water should feel comfortably warm to your elbow. If you use a bath thermometer aim for a temperature of 36.5–38°C (98–100°F).

3. Lie your baby on the changing mat, undress him down to his nappy and wrap him snugly in a towel spread across your knees.

4. Gently wash his eyelids, using a piece of cotton wool or cotton wool ball for each and wiping from the inside out.

5. His nose and ears are self-cleaning, so all you need to do is wipe off any obvious mucus or wax that is on the outside. Never insert a cotton bud or cotton wool in his nostrils or ears.

6. Wipe the rest of his face and gently pat him dry.

7. Now wash your baby's hair using baby soap, baby shampoo or an all-in-one bath liquid. Don't be afraid to wash the soft spots (fontanelles) at the front and back of his head, as they are protected by a tough membrane. Rinse his head thoroughly and dry gently.

8. Unwrap your baby and take off his nappy. Remove any soiling with soap and water, baby wipes or baby lotion, wiping from front to back if your baby is a girl.

9. Now lift your baby gently into the bath. Support his upper arm with one hand and his thigh with the other. Talk to him softly and reassuringly as he enters the water.

10. Holding his upper arm to stop him slipping into the water, wash and rinse his body with your other hand.

11. Lift him out of the bath and wrap him in his towel. Gently does it – he's as slippery as an eel!

12. Carefully pat him dry, paying special attention to the creases of his neck, thighs and bottom to ensure that he doesn't get sore. If you like you can dust a little baby powder over his body to make him smell nice.

13. Dress him in his clean, warm clothes and give him a hug.

Never leave the baby alone in the bath even for a second – he can drown in just 5 cm (2 in.) of water.

The first few times you bath your baby you will probably feel awkward. Bathing a real live baby, who seems to have suddenly sprouted twice as many arms and legs, all of them slippery, is very different from practising on a doll. Don't worry – it will soon become second nature.

Where shall I bath my baby?

You don't need to bath your baby in the bathroom. The bedroom, sitting room or even the kitchen are all suitable – whichever is most convenient. Room temperature should be about 21°C (70°F) and the windows should be closed to prevent your baby from becoming chilled.

You can bath him in a sink or wash-basin (wrap the taps in a piece of soft towel to prevent him from injury or burns), in a special baby bath, or even in a large plastic washing-up bowl. A special baby bath is handy if you can afford it, but your baby will soon outgrow it.

When shall I bath my baby?

There's no need to have a set bathtime in the early weeks. Choose a time when your baby is awake and happy or when it is convenient for you. It could be the middle of the morning, or perhaps at a time when he won't settle and you are at a loss to know what to do with him. As he gets older he will enjoy his bath as part of the bedtime routine. The warmth of the water will help to relax him ready for sleep.

At first it is a good idea to bath him after his feed, when he isn't hungry and irritable. If he is in the habit of going straight to sleep after a feed you could bath him halfway through the feed, before putting him to sleep.

What you need for bathtime

- Baby bath and stand, or large washing-up bowl
- Baby soap, baby shampoo or liquid bath solution
- Baby wipes or baby lotion
- Flannel
- Cotton wool or cotton wool balls
- Clean nappy and liner
- Waterproof pants
- Clean stretch suit or nightie
- Clean vest
- Large soft towel or bathrobe
- Changing mat

As your baby gets older

From the age of about four to six months, or when your baby can sit up on his own, he will be able to use the big bath. At first he may feel a bit daunted by the size. You can help him become used to it by placing his baby bath inside the big bath on the first few occasions. Once he is ready for the big bath, place a rubber mat or towel on the bottom of it to prevent him from slipping. If he is unable to sit up on his own, you'll need to support his back.

Topping and tailing

On the days you don't bath your baby, or every day if he dislikes being bathed, you can top and tail him. This means washing just the parts that are dirty.

STEP BY STEP TO TOPPING AND TAILING

1. Lay your baby on a folded towel, changing mat or any other convenient surface.
2. Collect together all the things you need (see below).
3. Take a piece of cotton wool, dip it in warm, boiled water and gently wipe one eye, from the bridge of his nose outwards. Using a fresh piece of cotton wool, do the same for the other eye.
4. Take another piece of cotton wool, dip it in water and clean the rest of his face and neck, being especially careful to wash in the folds of his skin where milk may have dribbled. Gently dry his face with a towel.
5. Wash his hands with a flannel and dry with a towel.
6. Take off his nappy and cleanse his bottom.
7. Put on clean nappy and clothes.

What you need for topping and tailing

- Changing mat or old, clean towel
- Towel
- Bowl of warm, boiled water
- Cotton wool or cotton wool balls
- Flannel
- Clean nappy and liner
- Waterproof pants
- Baby cream

HOW TO KEEP YOUR BABY CLEAN

• *Ears* and *nose* Your baby's ears and nose are self-cleaning. Don't attempt to clean them with a cotton wool bud, as this could damage the delicate tissues. Wipe away any excess mucus or wax from the outside of his nose or ears, using a piece of twisted cotton wool or cotton wool bud, and leave the inside to take care of itself.

• *Genitals* You need to clean your baby's genitals only on the outside. Never force back a baby boy's foreskin to clean underneath it as you could damage the delicate tissues there. The foreskin is normally attached to the tip of the penis, and will retract of its own accord over the next few years. Always wipe your baby girl's bottom from front to back to prevent bacteria from stools entering her bladder or vagina.

• *Hair* In the early days hair washing can be part of your baby's bath or topping and tailing routine. Use a mild baby shampoo, liquid bath solution or baby soap. By the time your baby is three months old he can have his hair rinsed with plain water daily, and a proper shampoo twice a week.

• *Nails* Even a newborn baby's fingernails may be long enough to scratch. Use special baby nail scissors or baby nail clippers. Some mothers find it easier to bite the baby's nails to trim them. Cut fingernails to a slightly rounded shape so there are no sharp edges; cut toenails straight across. If your baby wriggles too much, try doing it when he's asleep.

• *Navel* There is no need to wait for your baby's navel to heal before you give him a bath. The midwife will give you some surgical spirit or a special solution and show you how to clean his cord stump. Make sure you dry it completely after bathing, and powder it well.

My baby hates having his hair washed!

Take heart – you're not alone. The following tips may help tide you over until your baby becomes more co-operative:

• Stop hair washing for a few days to encourage him to forget he dislikes it. Wipe off any dust, dirt or bits of food with a damp flannel.
• Use a special non-stinging shampoo.
• Buy a headband to protect your baby's face during hair washing.
• When rinsing, hold his head back so that the water doesn't trickle on to his face, or simply wipe off the suds with a sponge or flannel wrung out in fresh water.

• *Skin* There's no need to do more than wash your baby's skin with soap or an all-in-one bath solution, then pat it gently dry, making sure you dry in the creases. Talc is not essential, but it is pleasant to rub on a little after your baby's bath. Alternatively your baby may enjoy being massaged with a mild oil such as almond, or baby oil.

EVERYTHING YOU NEED TO KNOW ABOUT NAPPIES

It is certain that over the next couple of years or so you will be spending a great deal of time changing nappies. The choice of nappies is between disposable and fabric (see page 19), but whichever type you choose the basic nappy-changing routine is the same.

Nappy-changing – when and where
• Change your baby's nappy whenever he is dirty or seems uncomfortable. In the early days that means every time you feed him, as a reflex action causes him to soil his nappy when he feeds.
• You may find it convenient, when breast-feeding, to change his nappy between sides. If he is inclined to drop off to sleep, this will have the advantage of waking him up sufficiently to take the second side. It also means you can put him straight to sleep after the feed.
• Change him in his pram or cot, on a changing mat, table or any convenient surface.
• Once your baby starts to roll it is safer to change him on the floor.

How to change your baby's nappy
1. Unbutton the lower part of his stretch suit.
2. Take off his plastic pants.
3. Unpin the nappy and use the corner to wipe away any excess soiling.
4. Lift your baby off the nappy and put it to one side.
5. Clean your baby's bottom using baby lotion and cotton wool, soap and water or baby wipes. Make sure that you wipe away all traces of bowel motion from the creases or he could become sore. You will probably need to use several swabs of cotton wool. Smear on a little baby cream.
6. Put on a clean nappy (see p. 22).
7. If he has wet or soiled his clothes remove and change.

8. Put your baby somewhere safe while you place the disposable nappy in a plastic bag and wash your hands.
9. If using a fabric nappy, flush liner down the lavatory and flush away soiling before putting the nappy in a sterilizing bucket.

What you need for nappy-changing

- Changing mat
- Clean disposable nappy, or fabric nappy with pins and liner
- Cotton wool or cotton wool balls
- Baby lotion, baby wipes or bowl of warm water and soap
- Cream
- Two sterilizing buckets for fabric nappies
- Plastic rubbish bag for soiled disposable nappies

The choice is finally up to you. You will need to take into account your lifestyle and circumstances, including whether you have facilities for easy washing and drying, and the state of your finances. Talk to other people who have children to find out their ideas and opinions.

Disposable nappies

Buying disposable nappies in bulk can save you money and the worry of running out of them at an inconvenient time. Several firms offer a door-to-door delivery service to save you carrying home bulky packs.

Despite manufacturers' claims, disposables can block up the drains if you flush them down the lavatory, so it is best to burn them or collect them in a plastic rubbish sack and put them in the dustbin.

What sort of disposable?

Mothers today have a bewildering assortment of disposable nappies to choose from. Disposable nappies usually come in three sizes – for babies up to 10 or 11 pounds, up to around 20 pounds and over 20 pounds – though some manufacturers offer additional sizes for newborns and older children. However, the weight of your child is only a rough guide, since babies come in all shapes and sizes. The various brands of nappy vary a lot in actual shape and size, so it's a question of trial and error which fits best.

Absorbency used to be a major problem in the early days of disposable nappies. Today's 'super' nappies have solved the problem of leaking once and for all. Instead of being made with a filling of

Disposable or fabric nappies – which should you choose?

Disposable nappies
Pros
- Convenient.
- Easy when you are out and about.
- Time-saving.
- Look neat under clothes.
- Little equipment needed.
- Convenient if your baby has nappy rash as you can change them often.
- Easy to change if space is at a premium.

Cons
- Expensive.
- Not reusable so you need to make sure you have a sufficient quantity.
- May leak.
- Tapes may come unstuck, although most varieties now have resealable tapes.
- Bulky to store and transport home from shops.
- Don't flush away easily.

Fabric nappies
Pros
- Cheap in the long run.
- May last over several babies.
- May need changing less often.
- Can be folded to fit any shape or size of baby.
- Can be used as cleaning cloths or dusters once their nappy days are over.

Cons
- Nappy washing is tedious and time-consuming.
- A great deal of other equipment is also needed, such as pins, plastic pants, sterilizing buckets, and so on.
- Awkward and messy when you are out.
- Nappy buckets in the bathroom.
- Become coarse with age.
- Look bulky and droopy under clothing.

woodpulp, the new nappies have a special powder in the middle which combines with the urine to form a gel, and is capable of holding about 800 times its own weight in water!

The very latest environment-friendly nappies are less sparkling in colour than the usual type of disposable. That's because they are not bleached with harsh chemicals – better for the rivers that these bleaches used to be washed into, and better for your baby's bottom too!

All disposables have elasticated legs to prevent leakage, but some brands have three or four separate rows of elastic, while others have a wider band of gathers. It doesn't really matter which you choose, but the nappy should fit closely around the leg. Some brands have a leakproof waistband too.

Most brands have resealable tapes, so you can undo the nappy and fasten it again as often as you like. Once your baby is on the move you'll appreciate this feature. Incidentally don't let any cream or powder come into contact with the tapes or they won't stick.

Several nappies have wetness indicators, motifs printed in water-soluble ink that dissolve and disappear when your baby has wet himself.

Prices of disposables vary a lot, but in general the bigger the pack the cheaper the nappy, so it's probably worth buying in bulk.

Fabric nappies

Most manufacturers make a range of nappies that vary in quality and absorbency. Buy the very best you can afford – you will need about 25. If you can't run to the highest quality look out for sales and seconds. The cheaper, unbranded sorts are often smaller, thinner and more likely to fray or wear into holes.

Muslin nappies are less absorbent but are soft and will fit snugly in the early months. Afterwards they make useful bibs or cloths.

Nappy liners

The one-way liners allow moisture to seep through to the nappy and so keep your baby's bottom dry, a boon if he is prone to nappy rash. Some nappy liners are intended to be laundered. You can also wash the ordinary disposable sort a couple of times before they disintegrate.

Plastic pants

You will need about six pairs of plastic pants, and there is a wide variety from which to choose. Pull-on ones are convenient and may help your baby stay dry better. Snap-on ones are handy to put on and allow the air to circulate. The tie-on variety often fit more neatly on a tiny baby. Pants made from waterproofed fabric are more expensive but will last longer and are kinder on a baby's skin than the traditional plastic ones, which tend to become brittle with constant washing.

Washing and sterilizing fabric nappies

You will need two sterilizing buckets and a supply of sterilizing powder or liquid. Make up fresh sterilizing solution every day. If your baby has soiled his nappy, dispose of the liner and rinse off any residue of soiling under the lavatory flush. Then put the nappy into the bucket that you keep for soiled nappies. If he has simply wet himself, nappy and liner can be put in the other bucket. Leave nappies in the sterilizing solution for the recommended time.

It is important to wash fabric nappies thoroughly to prevent the growth of germs that could cause nappy rash. Nappies that were just wet can be put through the rinse cycle of your washing machine, or rinsed thoroughly by hand. Soiled nappies should be washed in hot water with a gentle soap powder. There are several automatic washing powders on the market, which are specially designed for use with delicate fabrics. Avoid harsh biological detergents for a baby's washing.

Nappies can be dried in a tumble dryer, which will keep them soft and fluffy. Give them an occasional blow on the line in the open air, to help keep them white and kill off any lingering bacteria. Don't dry nappies over a radiator or heater, as it makes them coarse.

Tips for easy nappy-changing

- Fold a day's worth of fabric nappies ready for use.
- Keep a supply of nappy-changing equipment upstairs and down, so you can change your baby wherever he is.
- At night, use a double nappy or put a disposable pad inside a fabric nappy. Then if your baby only wets himself there is no need to change him until the morning.
- Keep two sterilizing buckets in the baby's room – one for soiled and the other for wet nappies.
- Buy Vaseline or zinc and castor oil cream, which are inexpensive and just as good as proprietary baby creams.
- If your baby's nappies leak try putting him in a larger pair of plastic pants.

HOW TO FOLD A NAPPY

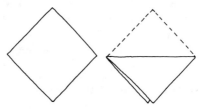

Triangle method
Fold the nappy in half diagonally so as to form a triangle. Bring the centre point up between the baby's legs and pin all three points

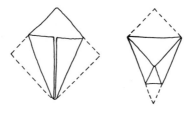

Kite method
Lay the nappy out so it forms a diamond. Bring two sides up to the middle. Fold down the top point to the centre and bring the bottom

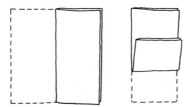

Rectangle method
Fold the nappy in half so that it forms a long rectangle. Fold down the top third for thickness at the back (for a girl), or the bottom third up for

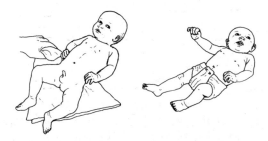

together in the middle. You can tuck the two ends under the baby's legs as you fold it, if you like, for a neater fit.

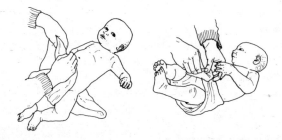

point up. Lie the baby on the nappy. Then bring up the bottom part and pin at each hip.

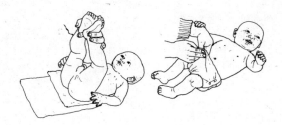

thickness at the front (for a boy). Pin at the sides with two safety pins.

Caring for plastic pants

Wash plastic pants by hand in warm water with a liquid soap or soap flakes. Machine-washing makes them brittle, as does washing in very hot or cold water. Pat them dry and leave to air, or hang them on the line.

Nappy rash

Most babies develop a sore bottom at some time or another. The soreness can vary from a slight redness to a serious rash with open sores. Nappy rash is distressing for your baby. With careful hygiene you should be able to prevent it or clear it up quickly if it starts to develop.

To prevent nappy rash

- Change your baby's nappy frequently, and always as soon as you know he has soiled it.
- Be especially careful over sterilizing and washing nappies.
- Use one-way nappy liners to keep his bottom dry.
- Clean his bottom thoroughly at every change.
- Leave him to kick without his nappy from time to time.
- Use pants made from waterproofed material to allow the air to get to his bottom, or better still leave them off altogether.

If your baby has nappy rash

- Leave your baby's nappy off so the air can heal the soreness. Lay him on a towel in his cot or pram, making sure you remove it the moment it is wet or soiled.
- Apply a special medicated cream to the affected area. Your health visitor, doctor or chemist will recommend one.
- Leave off his plastic plants.
- Use lotion rather than soap and water to clean his bottom.
- If the rash doesn't clear up using these simple measures consult your doctor as the baby could have an infection that needs treatment.

DRESSING YOUR BABY

Dressing your baby and deciding what to clothe him in is one of the delights of parenthood, especially with such a wide choice of bright, colourful and well-designed clothes on the market.

At first your baby will need changing quite frequently as he may dribble or posset, or his nappy may leak. Keep clothes simple and avoid too many buttons and fiddly fastenings: a wobbly newborn is quite difficult to dress until you get used to it.

Until your baby is able to support his neck and you are used to handling him, dress and undress him on a firm surface such as the bed, the sofa or the floor. Protect the surface with a changing mat and spread a towel on top to make it softer for your baby.

Tips on dressing

- Avoid clothes with too many ribbons, buttons or other fiddly fastenings.
- Choose all-in-one suits that are simple to get on and off.
- Avoid open-weave garments in which he could snag his fingers.
- Don't buy too many first-size clothes – he will grow out of them quickly.
- Avoid garments that fasten at the back.
- Buy vests with envelope necks or the sort that fasten at the front.
- Try not to cover your baby's face with the garment as you draw it over his head otherwise he will scream with panic.
- If you are buying separates make sure they cover his tummy – any gap between top and bottom will make him feel cold.
- Keep a careful check on the feet of all-in-one suits – as your baby grows his feet could become constricted. If the garment fits but the feet are too small, cut them off and use bootees or socks.
- Buy clothes that are easy to care for.

Clothes for a newborn baby

The following are a few suggestions for a basic wardrobe. Precisely what you buy will be dictated by your washing and drying facilities and your budget.

- 4–6 wide-necked cotton vests
- 4–6 all-in-one stretch suits or nighties
- 3 cardigans
- Coat or jacket, or for a winter baby an all-in-one quilted pram suit
- Hat and mittens
- Carrying shawls
- Sun hat and parasol for a summer baby

CARRYING YOUR BABY

Although your baby seems fragile he is quite hardy. However, until he can support his own head, you need to make sure it doesn't flop when you pick him up. Wrapping him in a shawl or swaddling him (see pages 56–7) will help him to feel secure and make him easier to carry around.

You can carry your baby in the traditional 'rock-a-bye-baby' way, or you can support him against your shoulder. Alternatively, you may find it easier to carry him in a sling or carrier (one with head support for a newborn baby), or baby nest.

An older baby can be carried astride your hips or facing outwards. He, too, will enjoy being carried in a sling – so long as your back can stand it! – or a backpack-type baby carrier.

Part II

FEEDING

BREAST-FEEDING

Coming home

It's exciting coming home with your new baby but it can also be worrying. All of a sudden you have total responsibility for your tiny newborn. However, breast-feeding is often easier at home than in hospital. You can feed your baby whenever appropriate, without the restrictions of ward routines and visiting times. Night feeds are easier, too, with no worries about waking other mothers or babies, and if your baby sleeps next to your bed you can simply lift her out and put her to the breast. Now you and your baby can really begin to get to know each other.

However, even though your baby may have seemed settled in hospital, the return home often sparks off bouts of unpredictable behaviour. You may lay the blame for this on your milk supply. Try not to worry as it will only make matters worse. It takes several weeks for a baby to settle into a regular routine. Stay calm and relaxed and by the time your baby is six weeks old you will probably find that all the early problems have sorted themselves out, and you can begin to enjoy the very real advantages of breast-feeding.

How to cope with breast-feeding when you come home

- If your baby seems unsettled don't blame your milk supply – it is simply that she is sensitive to any change in her surroundings.
- Keep the pram or carrycot downstairs so you don't have so much running around to do.
- Rest as much as possible and don't entertain too many visitors.
- Employ help in the home if you can afford it, or find out from your health visitor if you are eligible for a local authority home help.
- Simplify life as much as you can while you establish a routine – for instance, don't worry about getting housework done, keep meals simple, etc.
- Night feeds may be easier if you have your baby sleeping in your room.
- Have a drink and snack ready before starting to breast-feed.
- Make sure the room is warm enough – about 21°C (70°F).
- Keep a supply of baby clothes and nappies downstairs to save having to collect them from upstairs at every feed time.
- Always find a comfortable place in which to sit before starting to feed – and take the opportunity to put your feet up.

BREAST-FEEDING PROBLEMS

Problem	Symptoms
Leaky breasts	Milk leaks from the breasts during and between feeds.
Refusal to suck	Baby arches her back and strains away from the breast even though you know she must be hungry. She appears to fight the breast.

Cause	Solution
Supply and demand not yet settled down.	Wear thick, non-plastic-backed pads in your bra to soak up leaks, or try one-way nappy liners or folded men's hankies. Frequent changes of bra and nightclothes. Leaking stops when supply and demand have adjusted.
Pressure on breasts during the night from the way you are lying.	Feed baby immediately before going to bed. Protect bedclothes with a towel.
Breasts release milk when you are not feeding (let-down reflex).	Press firmly against your nipples until you feel the tingling ease.
Baby's nose blocked either by a cold or by over-full breasts.	If baby has a cold ask your doctor whether he or she recommends nose drops. Hold baby more upright when feeding. Support breast from underneath so that baby's nostrils are clear.
Baby panics when offered the breast, perhaps initially as a result of above, and a habit has set in.	Stay calm. Experiment with different feeding positions, e.g. with her body tucked under your arm, standing up, lying down, and so on. Pick up your baby and put her to the breast while she is sleepy, before she has the chance to know what is happening.
Baby prefers one side.	Start feeding on the side she prefers least, so that she is hungry when she takes it. Move baby across to the other breast, keeping her in the same position when you change sides, i.e. so that her feet are under your arm.

BREAST-FEEDING PROBLEMS

Problem	Symptoms
Sleepy baby	Baby falls asleep during feed and can't be aroused. Baby fails to wake and demand feeds.
Apparently low milk supply	Baby not gaining or losing weight. Scanty, dry stools. Dry or only dampish nappy. No milk flow (let-down reflex). Baby fractious and irritable.

Cause	Solution
Pain-relieving drugs are still circulating in her system, making her sleepy, or you are taking medication, e.g. tranquillizers, which are passed on via the milk.	Be patient and persevere, the problem will ease as the drugs pass out of her system. In the meantime, wake her for at least six feeds a day. If she drops off to sleep try removing some of her clothing to arouse her. Hold her in a more upright position, change her nappy. If the problem is caused by prescribed medication, ask the doctor whether another drug could be substituted. Keep a careful check on your baby's weight gain.
Baby is unwell.	If baby is extremely sleepy and hard to arouse, consult your doctor.
Surroundings are too hot.	Open a window.
Temporary imbalance between supply and demand.	Feed baby more frequently. Rest and relax, and step up your calorie intake. Avoid complementary bottles as they can further reduce supply. Check with your doctor that baby is not ill.
Baby not on breast properly, so failing to spark off let-down reflex.	Check position. The nipple and the area around it should be well in your baby's mouth. Remove excess clothing so baby has free access to your breast and nipple. Watch to see the muscles at the side of her ears working to check she's on correctly.
Anxiety	Relax and breathe deeply when you feed.
Baby being given top-up bottles so weakening strength of her sucking.	Cut out top-ups from the bottle and boost milk supply as described above.
Baby in need of a bit of company. Naturally fretful baby. Your anxiety and inexperience.	Keep cot downstairs, pick your baby up and cuddle her. Carry her around with you in a sling as you go about your chores. Follow tips in chapter on crying and sleep. Have confidence in yourself. This is your baby and you know best. Get genned up on breast-feeding, or contact a breast-feeding self-help group.

BREAST-FEEDING PROBLEMS

Problem	Symptoms
Apparently low milk supply	Baby not gaining or losing weight. Scanty, dry stools. Dry or only dampish nappy. No milk flow (let-down reflex). Baby fractious and irritable.
Blocked milk duct	Tender and sore red lump. Flu-like feeling.
Mastitis	Same as above, except feverish symptoms more marked and pain over hardened areas of the breast.
Baby gaining excessive amount of weight (280–450 g/10–16 oz.).	

Looking after yourself

A happy, relaxed mother usually makes for a contented baby, so it is important to take care of yourself when you are breast-feeding. When a mother is convinced that she hasn't enough milk, the reason is often that the milk is not being released. Breast milk is stored in special glands deep inside the breasts. When your baby sucks at the breast, hormones are released that cause the milk to be propelled down the milk channels and out through the nipples. This is called the let-down

Cause	Solution
Tight clothing or bra cutting into your breast and preventing free flow along milk ducts.	Don't wear tight clothing and buy a well-fitting special nursing bra. For a few feeds offer sore breast first to allow baby's hungry sucking to drain breast. Gently massage above and below lump to get milk moving. Apply hot or cold compresses for relief
Milk build-up as a result of breast being insufficiently emptied.	Give extra feeds to keep breast as empty as possible.
Untreated blocked duct causing milk to seep into surrounding tissue.	Continue treatment as above and consult your doctor, who will probably prescribe antibiotics to prevent an infection developing.
Infection caused by bacteria from baby's nose getting into milk. Laboratory tests will confirm presence of bacteria.	Continue treatments as for blocked duct. Rest and have plenty to drink. Consult your doctor; if mastitis is left untreated at this stage it could progress to an abscess that has to be surgically drained.
Misinterpretation of baby's signals, such as crying, fretfulness, and so on, as always meaning hunger.	Cut feeds to five or six a day, and try other ways of comforting her, such as using a dummy, or any of the methods suggested in the chapter on crying (see pages 54–7).
Sometimes a baby gains large amounts of weight for no apparent reason.	If you are already giving only five or six feeds a day continue as before. Your baby's weight gain may even out once she starts to eat solids and become more active.

reflex – you may notice it as a strong, pricking sensation when you start feeding and may see milk shooting in fine jets or dripping steadily from your nipples. The reflex can be triggered off by your baby feeding, or even by just thinking about your baby; but it can also be suppressed if you are tense or anxious. So you can see that if you worry about not producing enough milk, a vicious circle can be formed.

Breast-feeding makes demands on your body's food reserves, so it is important that you eat well, too. Your body laid down stores of fat during pregnancy for this purpose, and changes in the rate at which your body burns up food during breast-feeding should ensure that you are able to provide for your baby. You may find that you produce a better milk supply if you have about 500 extra calories a day, so eat a wholesome snack mid-morning and mid-afternoon. If you are usually of normal weight, it is unwise to diet when you are breast-feeding. If you are very overweight a sensible diet should do no harm – ask your health visitor for advice.

Like any new skill, breast-feeding takes a while to learn, and you may encounter one or two difficulties in the early weeks. The chart shows some of the most common problems, which may look daunting, but you are unlikely to experience all of them – unless you are exceptionally unlucky. If you do have breast-feeding problems ask for help and advice from your health visitor, doctor, or one of the mother-to-mother support groups listed on page 139.

Growth spurts

Your baby will gain weight in fits and starts. So long as she is gaining weight and seems contented, and your health visitor is happy with her progress, there is no need to worry about the amount of weight she puts on. Most of the average weight gains given in books are based on those of artificially fed babies. Having your baby weighed regularly at the clinic will help to reassure you that you are doing your best for your baby, or you can weigh your baby at home by stepping on to the scales and weighing yourself accurately and then stepping on holding your baby.

Your milk production works by supply and demand, so that every so often, as your baby takes a leap in growth, her needs will temporarily outstrip your supply. Such growth spurts, as they are called, are quite easily dealt with. Your baby will usually demand to be fed more often for a day or so; and because the more often you feed, the more milk you will make, your supply will soon catch up with her demand. If her weight stays still for several weeks, or she actually loses weight but doesn't ask for extra feeds, try stepping up the number of feeds you offer, and follow the measures suggested on page 33 for building up your milk supply.

Growth spurts commonly happen at the age of six weeks, 12 weeks and four to six months, but they can also occur at any other time.

When should I stop breast-feeding?

There's no easy answer to this question, because so much depends on your personal lifestyle and circumstances. If you are going back to work, at around seven months after birth, you may want to accustom your baby to having a bottle, so that the person who is looking after her can feed her. Alternatively, you may like to continue giving one or two breast-feeds a day, say before you go to work and when you come home, or you may be prepared to express breast milk to be fed to her by bottle while you are away. If you opt to express breast milk you will need somewhere private to do this during working hours, and a fridge in which to store the milk. Ask your health visitor or one of the breast-feeding self-help groups (see page 139) for advice.

You may aim to breast-feed until your baby is well established on solids (see page 46), and then, if your baby likes sucking – and most babies do up to a year – gradually substitute milk from a cup or a bottle. Alternatively, you may want to breast-feed for longer than the first year. There is no reason why you shouldn't so long as you and your baby are happy with it.

Some babies give up feeding of their own accord, others need help to persuade them to stop.

Whatever you decide is right for you and your baby, proceed slowly, always leaving two or three days at least between dropping each feed, to give your breasts time to adjust to the reduced demand. The process of weaning to solids usually takes place over two or three months.

If you are weaning a baby under three months on to a bottle the following schedule is practical and should enable both you and your baby to become used to the change in feeding method. If your breasts feel uncomfortable slow down the schedule to give them time to adjust.

Weaning to a bottle – suggested weaning schedule

DAY ONE 5 breast-feeds	1 bottle-feed
DAY TWO 5 breast-feeds	1 bottle-feed
DAYS THREE AND FOUR 4 breast-feeds	2 bottle-feeds
DAYS FIVE TO SEVEN 3 breast-feeds	3 bottle-feeds
DAYS EIGHT AND NINE 2 breast-feeds	4 bottle-feeds
DAYS TEN TO FOURTEEN 1 breast-feed	5 bottle-feeds
AFTER THAT	6 bottle-feeds

BOTTLE-FEEDING

There's no doubt that breast is best for your baby. But if you opt to bottle-feed for whatever reason don't let feelings of guilt that you aren't breast-feeding mar what should be an enjoyable experience. Babies fed on the bottle thrive quite happily, and so long as you observe a few hygiene rules, bottle-feeding is perfectly safe.

One advantage of bottle-feeding is that people other than his mother can give the feed, which gives you the occasional break and your baby the opportunity to form relationships with other people. Nonetheless, you and his father should aim to give most of your baby's feeds.

Cuddle your baby close when you feed him, and make feed times pleasant, social occasions. Don't ever leave your baby propped up alone with his bottle. Not only will he be lonely, but there is a very real danger that he could choke.

Type of formula	Ingredients	Suitable for
Highly modified or humanized milk	Skimmed cow's milk, whey, mixed fats, lactose	New baby, although it can be used throughout bottle-feeding. Most useful if you want to demand feed your baby, because it is easily digested and absorbed.
Modified skimmed milk	Skimmed cow's milk, fats, lactose or maltodextrin	New baby or from a few weeks. Maltodextrin stays longer in the baby's system than lactose, so he may demand to be fed less frequently.
Modified whole milk	Whole cow's milk, lactose or maltodextrin, or a mixture of the two	For the hungrier baby. Baby may settle into a routine more readily because of fat content and effect of sugar on his appetite-control mechanism.
Milk-free formula	Vegetable oil and soya protein	If your baby is allergic to cow's milk. Should be given on medical advice only.

Which milks?

There is a bewildering choice of baby milks on the market; and, as the manufacturers discover more about the precise make-up of breast milk, new formulas are brought out to mimic it more closely. Most baby milks are made from modified cow's milk, with fats and sugars added. The type of sugar varies from one milk to another. Some contain only lactose, the special milk sugar that is known to be contained in breast milk. Others contain a sort of sugar called maltodextrin, which may give your baby a greater feeling of satisfaction, so that his appetite-regulating mechanism is suppressed for longer. Your health visitor will advise you on the most suitable milk for your baby, and the chart below will help you appreciate the different types.

Feeding your baby

In the early days your baby will thrive best if you feed him on demand, as you would a breast-fed baby. You can do this quite easily by making up a whole day's supply of milk and keeping it in the fridge. While your baby is having more than four to six feeds a day, you may find it easier to make up the supply in a couple of batches, to avoid having to buy extra bottles of sterilizing equipment.

Warming the bottle

Milk doesn't need to be warmed, but you may feel a warm feed is more comforting for your baby. To warm, take the bottle of feed out of the fridge and place it in a jug of hot water, to bring the contents to blood heat. Test the temperature by first shaking the bottle and then letting a couple of drops fall on to your wrist. It should feel the same temperature as your skin.

Running the bottle under the hot tap will warm it quickly. You can also use a special bottle warmer. Do not warm feed in the microwave, as the milk in the middle of the bottle can become very hot and scald the baby.

You should never store milk that has been warmed, keep it in a thermos flask, or leave it standing for any length of time in a bottle warmer, as germs grow rapidly in warm milk. Always discard any unused milk after your baby has had his feed.

Milk flow

The milk should flow out of the teat in a steady stream of several drips per second when you hold the bottle upside down. The traditional latex teats may need to have the hole enlarged from time to time by using a sterilized needle or making a sharp cross-shaped cut with a razor blade, and the teats need to be replaced every couple of months as the rubber starts to wear.

Transparent silicone teats are easier to clean and need replacing less often than the traditional type of teat.

A new baby needs a teat with a slow rate of flow. Choose 'slow', 'small' or 'newborn' sizes, progressing to medium and large as your baby grows and his sucking becomes more vigorous.

There have been reports of babies choking on dummies made from silicone as a result of chewing off fragments of teat. This is unlikely to happen with a bottle teat, as the baby spends less time chewing on it than he would a dummy. However, keep an eye on the teat, and replace any that have become punctured.

Hygiene

Scrupulous hygiene is essential when you are bottle-feeding. All bottles, teats and feeding equipment should be sterilized until your baby is at least six months old. There are several methods of sterilizing. The old-fashioned method of boiling involves thoroughly cleaning the teats and bottles, then putting them into a saucepan and boiling for five minutes, making sure that there are no air bubbles.

Until recently, the easiest way to sterilize was to use a chemical sterilizing solution, or tablets in a sterilizing unit or other covered plastic container.

A special steam sterilizer is the latest alternative method. The bottles are simply placed in the sterilizer with a small amount of water. The appliance is switched on and after five minutes it switches itself off and the bottles are sterilized. The cost of this unit works out at about the same as a chemical sterilizing kit and a year's supply of solution or tablets.

Coping with night feeds

Night feeds demand a little more forethought when you are bottle-feeding, as you can't simply pick up the baby and put him on the breast. However, with a bit of forward planning you can keep any disturbance to the minimum. Pack two made-up bottles from the fridge into an insulated bag or box. Take a vacuum flask of hot water and a jug or bowl, or a bottle warmer, in which to warm the bottle. Your baby won't sleep through the night before he weighs 280 g (10 lb.), but after that you could try and encourage him to wait longer between feeds. Make any change gradually. Bring the baby's late evening feed slowly forward by half an hour every couple of days, and at the same time pick him up half an hour later for his early morning feed. Hopefully this should enable you to snatch a few more hours' uninterrupted sleep.

How much does he need?
You can safely be guided by your baby's appetite. Today's bottle milks are so similar to breast milk that you can demand feed in much the same way as a breast-feeding mother.

Thirst
Bottle-fed babies get thirsty, especially in hot weather. If your baby seems to be hungry soon (less than two hours) after he has been fed try giving him a drink of cool, boiled water. After the age of a month he can have diluted orange or other fruit juice between feeds.

Overfeeding
To avoid overfeeding always let your baby decide when he's had enough. Don't force him to finish his bottle if he doesn't seem inclined, and never use more than the stated amount of milk powder when making up a feed. Not only can this make him fat, it could also put damaging strain on his kidneys.

Underfeeding
Very occasionally underfeeding is a problem for a bottle-fed baby. If your baby always downs his bottle and then looks around for more and he is also light in weight for his age, it could be that he isn't having enough feed. Make up an extra amount of baby milk. He's probably going through a growth spurt and needs an increased amount of milk. If your baby demands to be fed often but doesn't seem to take all his feed, check the teat. It could be that the hole is too small.

Possetting baby
Although some babies are naturally more prone than others to bring back a little milk after feeding (possetting), if your bottle-fed baby often regurgitates when he burps it could be that he is taking in too much air

with his bottle-feed. Check that the teat hole is large enough and make sure that the neck of the bottle is full of milk when you tilt it for him, to avoid his swallowing air as he takes his feed.

Constipation
Some babies pass a bowel motion every day, and others only once or twice a week. So long as the motion is soft it doesn't matter how often he opens his bowels.

If your baby's bowel motions are hard, dry and infrequent, and he has difficulty in passing them, he could be constipated. The reason is usually insufficient fluids. Give your baby plenty to drink, especially in hot weather. You can add an extra 30 ml (1 fl. oz.) of water to his bottle, and give him extra fruit drinks if he seems thirsty between feeds. A teaspoon or so of prune juice added to his water may help if the problem is severe. Never give your baby a laxative. If none of these remedies works consult your doctor.

INTRODUCING SOLIDS

Your baby will thrive well on milk from breast or bottle for the first four to six months of her life. From time to time she will undergo growth spurts, which you can deal with by increasing the amount of milk if you are bottle-feeding, or feeding more often for a day or so to build up your milk supply if you are breast-feeding.

However, some time between four and six months she may demand more feed but still seem to be unsatisfied. Now is the time to start thinking about introducing solids. If your baby doesn't seem keen, wait and try again a few months later.

There's no point in offering her solids before the age of four to six months, since her digestive system will not be able to cope with them, and physical and emotional problems may result if you try to start too early. Trying to force her to take solid food before she is ready will cause anxiety and frustration in both of you. It may also lead to fatness and arouse food allergies in your baby.

How to start
Stay relaxed and calm and make meal times fun. Avoid starting solids if

your baby is teething, unwell, or if she is experiencing other upsets or changes in her life.

To start off with, choose a time when your baby is happy and settled, for instance at lunch time. Let her have one breast, or half her bottle, to take the edge off her appetite. She'll be more willing to experiment if she's not ravenously hungry. At this stage your main aim is to persuade her to try different tastes and textures.

Sit your baby on your lap, take a small amount of sloppy food – for instance, mashed banana mixed with a little breast or bottle milk so it is very runny, broth, or puréed carrot – and gently put it to her lips. Use a small, flattish spoon, such as a coffee spoon or a special baby spoon, and don't push it too far into her mouth or she will choke. At first your baby won't know how to cope with this strange experience. She will probably spit the food out. Don't worry – it's not that she doesn't like it, just that she doesn't yet know what to do. At this stage, one spoonful is quite sufficient. Once she's had this first taste, continue with the rest of her milk feed.

Over the next few weeks offer a variety of different new tastes, allowing a couple of days between each new food to make sure it doesn't upset your baby. If she doesn't like a particular food, leave it and try it again a few days later. Bear in mind that, for the whole of her first year, milk is still her main form of nourishment. This way you are less likely to become upset and agitated if she doesn't like a particular food.

What food?
To begin with choose bland, puréed foods that are semi-liquid so she can suck them off the spoon. Gluten-free cereals, such as baby rice (wheat-based ones can set up allergies in susceptible babies), mashed or puréed fruits, root vegetables, cauliflower or broccoli, are all suitable. Don't give your baby oranges, grapefruit or other acid fruits or soft fruits, such as strawberries and raspberries, which have pips.

Moving on
Once your baby has become used to a wide range of tastes and textures, you can slowly step up the amount of food she has. The solid food can become the main part of her meal followed by a breast- or bottle-feed as a drink. Gradually add solids to the morning and evening feeds too, so that she moves towards a pattern of three meals a day.

How fast you proceed depends on your baby – the suggested schedule

below is for guidance only. Your baby may progress at a different rate
from this, which shouldn't worry you, as milk will form the mainstay of
her diet until she is a year old.

Finger foods

By the time your baby is six months old she will be able to chew,
whether or not she has teeth. She is also becoming adept at using her
hands – and everything goes to her mouth. You can exploit her
new-found skills by introducing a wider range of textures and one or
two finger foods with which she can feed herself. Babies who have not
been offered solid textures by the age of about nine months sometimes
take a long time to accept them. The way to avoid this problem is to
make the purées gradually more solid in texture. Mince or mash food,
and leave one or two soft lumps for her to chew.

Ringing the changes

You can also start mixing tastes and textures. Mashed banana can be
offered with cottage cheese, yoghurt or egg custard. Carrot can be used
with meat in a soup or stew.

Experiment with more unusual tastes too, for instance mashed
avocado pear, which some babies enjoy. However, steer clear of salted,
smoked or highly seasoned foods, and never add salt or sugar to your
baby's food.

Commercial baby foods

Commercial foods can save time when you are in a hurry, if you are out,
or if the rest of the family is having something which is unsuitable for a
baby. There is a wide range of tins and packets on the market. The
packet foods are especially useful in the early stages of weaning on to
solids, when your baby may be having only a teaspoonful or so of food.
The main disadvantage of commercial foods is that they tend to be
rather bland and smooth in texture. You will want your baby to join in
with family meals as soon as possible, so when she is aged between six
and nine months start offering her regular tastes of the food that the
rest of the family is eating. Bear in mind that when cooking your food
you will need to put a little of it aside for the baby before you add any
seasoning.

How to avoid meal-time misery

It is important that your baby enjoys her food and that meal time does not become a battleground. Stay calm at meal times and don't be upset if your baby doesn't like a particular food. It's the food she's rejecting, not you. You can't force a baby to eat, and by becoming engaged in meal-time battles you could be setting up a long-term problem that may prove exceptionally hard to overcome.

It's not vital for your baby to have any one particular food. Learn all about food values, and you will soon become expert at the art of substitution. For example, if she doesn't like milk, substitute cheese or yoghurt, which supply her with the same nutrients. If she doesn't like egg, mix it into puddings or a custard to disguise it.

Don't worry if your baby's meals seem unbalanced in the course of a day; a baby left to her own devices will take the nutrients she needs. When trying to balance your baby's food intake, try to think in terms of weeks rather than days.

Family meal times

Sit your baby from an early age at the table with the rest of the family, so she realizes that meal times are social occasions. Don't expect good manners to start with. Your baby will like to squash her food and explore it with her fingers and mouth. Put a stout bib on her and protect the floor with a plastic tablecloth. She'll get more civilized in her eating habits as she gets older and more adept at using her hands.

Don't expect your baby to sit at the table until everyone else has finished. About 20 minutes is as long as you can hope for at this age.

Encouraging independence

Give your baby a spoon at the age of about six months and let her try to feed herself. At first more food will go over her face than in her mouth, so you will have to do most of the feeding, but as she becomes more skilful she will start to feed herself. Provide her with a few finger foods at every meal; most babies prefer small servings to big platefuls. Make her food look attractive and colourful: bright portions of separate vegetables and meat look more appetizing than a brown mass.

Four to six months

Your baby is ready for a few early tastes. Don't add sugar to food. Very gradually introduce tiny tastes of a variety of simple foods. After a few

SUGGESTED WEANING SCHEDULE

First stage (four to six months and beyond)

On waking
Breast- or bottle-feed

Breakfast
Breast- or bottle-feed

Lunch time
Half breast- or bottle-feed followed by a couple of teaspoons of solid food, then rest of feed
Gradually increase the amount of solid food

Early evening
Breast- or bottle-feed

Bedtime
Breast- or bottle-feed

Second stage (six to eight months and beyond)

On waking
Breast- or bottle-feed

Breakfast
Baby cereal
Breast- or bottle-feed

Lunch time
Breast- or bottle-feed
Portion (one or two teaspoons) of rice with puréed vegetable
One teaspoon of puréed meat, fish, cottage cheese

Teatime
Slices of raw apple, carrot sticks and other finger foods

Early evening
Breast- or bottle-feed
Two teaspoons of cereal, tiny sandwiches or yoghurt and fruit

Bedtime
Breast- or bottle-feed

Third stage (eight months to a year)

On waking
Water or fruit juice

Breakfast
Cereal, hard-boiled or poached egg, bread or rusk with margarine or butter and smear of smooth peanut butter or yeast extract
Milk, water or fruit juice

Lunch time
Chopped or mashed fish, meat, pulses with lightly steamed or boiled vegetables
Milk pudding, fresh fruit, yoghurt, egg custard
Water or fruit juice

Teatime
Pieces of fresh fruit

Family meal time
Bread with savoury spread
Cucumber, carrot sticks, finger food
Jelly
Milk or apple juice

Bedtime
Breast- or bottle-feed or milk or milk drink made from baby milk or follow-on formula

weeks step up the amounts of foods. As your baby takes more solids gradually decrease the amount of bottle milk or the number of minutes on the breast. Don't force your baby to eat.

Finger foods

Finger foods help your baby to become independent and encourage her to chew rather than suck. Bear in mind that you should never leave your baby alone with finger foods in case she chokes.

The following are a few suggestions for finger foods. You'll think of others yourself – use your imagination!

- Sticks or cubes of vegetables and fruit, e.g. banana, apple, pear, cooked carrot, potatoes, cauliflower florets, bean sprouts, avocado
- Dried fruits, e.g. apricots, apples, peaches, dates, raisins
- Cubes of cheese
- Macaroni cheese
- Fingers of cheese on toast
- Rusks
- Puffed wheat, cornflakes, rice crispies (without milk poured over them)
- Cooked rice
- Miniature meatballs (home-made without seasoning)
- Cottage cheese
- Chunks of fish with bones removed
- Slices of hard-boiled egg
- Grated cheese
- Tiny sandwiches of smooth peanut butter or a savoury spread
- Smooth chicken bone with a few shreds of meat on it

Six to nine months

Your baby starts to feed herself. She also starts to chew. Start offering more coarsely textured foods, that is, minced and mashed rather than puréed. Make meals look attractive and appetizing. Mix colours and textures. Try giving her tastes of family meals, but avoid fried or spicy foods. As your baby's teeth come through, offer her a choice of hard foods such as raw apple or carrot. Always stay with her at such times so that you can ensure she doesn't choke. Start offering your baby drinks of water or diluted fruit juice from a feeder cup. You can encourage her to drink from an ordinary cup by occasionally offering her liquid from her feeder cup with the lid removed. You will need to help her with this, otherwise she will splash the drink over the floor.

Nine to twelve months

Your baby will now be feeding herself and you can include her in family meal times. Once she is happy drinking from a cup, you can gradually phase out her breast- or bottle-feeds altogether. However, if you want to continue with the odd feed or so into the second year there is no need to wean her completely so long as you are both happy. At about a year your baby still needs about 500 ml (1 pint) of milk a day.

---

10 tips for weaning without tears

- Take weaning slowly and gradually.
- Don't season or sweeten food and don't offer nuts or sweets.
- Cook meat and fish thoroughly and avoid reheating.
- Don't feed your baby direct from the jar unless she finishes the whole jar at a sitting. Her saliva could contaminate the food.
- Pay scrupulous attention to hygiene (but there's no need to sterilize when your baby is over six months old).
- Be guided on quantity of food by your baby's appetite. Her weight gain will start to slow down after the age of six months.
- Always make sure she is securely strapped in her highchair.
- Bear with any food fads or refusals cheerfully and calmly.
- Make food look attractive and colourful.
- Let your baby join in with family meal times as soon as possible, so that she sees meal times as happy, social occasions.

How to cope with feeding on holiday

- Try to keep as close as possible to your baby's normal feed times.
- Make sure you have a good supply of fruit drinks and water for the journey, in case she gets hot and thirsty.
- If you are travelling by air, put your baby to the breast or give her a drink from a bottle when you feel your ears start to pop as the plane descends. This way your baby may avoid discomfort.
- Take special care over hygiene and boil all water if you are holidaying in a hot climate.
- Take your usual brand of baby milk with you if you are travelling abroad – foreign varieties may vary slightly.

Solid feeding – what you need

- Two sizes of shallow spoon, for early solids and later on when she starts to feed herself. Your baby may find feeding herself is easier

What foods?

Fruit. Banana, peeled apple and pear (cooked for babies under six months), peeled plums, grapes, apricots with stones or pips removed, fresh or boiled in a little water. Avoid soft fruit with pips.

Vegetables. Puréed or grated carrot; once she's over six months, celery, cucumber, tomatoes, with seeds, skin and any coarse or stringy bits removed, can be given raw. Steamed or puréed peas, potatoes, spinach, beans, courgettes. Steer clear of sweetcorn, mushroom, onions at first. Delay introducing dried peas and beans (pulses) until she is past nine months. When you do introduce them, make sure they are thoroughly soaked and cooked, according to the directions on the packet.

Meat and fish. After six months, white meat such as chicken, grilled, roasted or stewed. As she gets used to solids introduce red meat and offal. White fish, steamed, grilled or baked. Avoid oily fish, tinned fish, smoked fish or shellfish.

Bread and cereals. Start off with rice, as some babies are allergic to the gluten in wheat products. From six months you can introduce wheat-based cereals, bread, macaroni and so on.

Milk and dairy products. From six months your baby can have baby milk, or a follow-on formula. By a year she can have unboiled cow's milk. If she doesn't like milk or is allergic to it consult your health visitor. If she doesn't like milk offer yoghurt, cottage cheese or mild hard cheese, or disguise it in puddings or custard.
Eggs. Some babies are allergic to egg white. Keep off it until she is eight or nine months old. Egg yolk should be hard-boiled, sieved and mixed to a suitable consistency with baby milk.

using a special 'bent' spoon that allows her to take the food into her mouth at the correct angle.
- Highchair, with harness to prevent your baby falling out.
- Different types of bib. The plastic-backed towelling type is most suitable for early days. Later on, use the sort with a trough that collects spilt food.
- Hand or electric food blender or grinder. You can purée or mash food by hand, but a special grinder or blender will make the job considerably easier.
- Unbreakable spouted cup. One with two handles is easier for your baby to manage than the single-handled variety.

- Unbreakable feeding bowl. Choose from bowls with a suction pad on the bottom to anchor them to the feeding tray; with space for a reservoir of warm water to keep your baby's food warm; and with a raised lip to prevent the food being pushed over the edge.

Part III

SLEEP AND CRYING

THE LANGUAGE OF CRYING

Babies cry because they can't talk and tell you what is wrong with them. There's nothing quite so powerful, or heart-rending, as hearing your baby cry. Try as you might to ignore the cries, it's impossible and you have to go to your baby. Your baby's cry is designed to agitate you. It's nature's way of ensuring that you care for him and protect him from harm.

A cry can mean: 'I'm hungry – come and feed me'; 'I'm tired now – let me sleep'; 'I'm bored – come and entertain me'; 'I'm lonely – I need your company'; 'I'm afraid – are you still there?' The problem for new parents is how to interpret their baby's message among all the myriad shades of meaning.

In some cultures babies are carried around all the time. When the mother needs a rest, she simply hands the baby over to someone else to hold for a while. Babies brought up in such communities are said to cry very rarely. It's hardly practical for most of us to carry our babies with us the whole time. Nevertheless, an almost certain way to soothe a fretful baby is to pick him up and hold him. You can't spoil your baby by doing this. In fact, research has shown over and over again that babies who are responded to the second they cry learn to trust those around them and fuss less than those who are left to cry long and loud before having their needs attended to.

Sometimes the reason your baby is crying is blindingly obvious (see table on page 58). At other times it seems impossible to work out what is bothering him. As you get to know him better, and as he increases his repertoire of expressions, you'll become more skilful at recognizing the meaning of his different cries. In the meantime it's a matter of trial and error. You won't always respond appropriately to his cries, but there will be times when you do and your baby will reward you with a huge, gummy smile.

How much your baby cries depends on his personality and how you handle him. Some babies are naturally fretful; others are more robust. It's easy to blame yourself if you have a baby who is inclined to be sensitive and grizzly, but try not to. A calm, unflustered approach will help you deal with his crying with more confidence, and your baby will come to realize that the world is not a place to be afraid of. As you get to know your baby, you will be able to handle him according to his individual temperament.

There may be times of the day when your baby seems more irritable than usual. Many babies cry more in the early evening. If your baby is among these, leave yourself time for him in the evening by making a few practical adjustments, such as preparing the family's evening meal earlier in the day.

How can I stop my baby crying?

So what can you do when your baby cries? Here are some tried-and-tested remedies.

Rocking This is a good way to soothe a restless baby and works best if you hold your baby in an upright position and jiggle him up and down at a rate of about 60–70 rocks a minute – the same rate as your pulse. Rocking your baby from side to side makes him lively. Rocking should be steady and continuous in order to be effective. The only limit is your patience – and the strength of your arms!

For the faint-hearted and weak-armed there are artificial aids available to rock your baby. One is a frame with a hammock attached, in which you place your baby's carrycot or Moses basket. A spring attached to the frame rocks the container up and down rhythmically. The other is a device that clips on to the pram handle and rocks it up and down.

Sound Any fairly loud, droning noise will soothe your baby until he is about four months old. The ticking of a clock, the whirr of a convector heater, the drone of a vacuum cleaner, or the vibrating of a washing machine or tumble dryer, has sent many a baby off to sleep! Rocking and sound combined is often a sure-fire soporific – which is perhaps why so many babies drop off to sleep in the car.

The traditional soothing sound is the lullaby. Try singing old favourites to him, such as 'Rock-A-Bye-Baby' and 'Bye Baby Bunting', or modern lullabies such as John Lennon's 'Beautiful Boy'.

If sound seems to settle your baby, you could try playing a soother tape to him. You can buy a tape of womb sounds, which have a quietening effect especially if you start to play it to him soon after birth.

Sucking Your new baby is a born sucker! He will often drift into sleep

Tips for using a dummy

- Use the dummy if your baby seems restless even though he has been fed, or at any time when you don't have time to spend rocking or soothing him in other ways. Some babies like to have a dummy to suck themselves to sleep.
- Don't give your baby a dummy simply for convenience. Watch out for signs that he is becoming restless, such as gnawing his hand or yawning.
- Always wash the dummy carefully after use and sterilize it until your baby is six months old.
- Don't put the dummy back in his mouth if it has fallen on the floor.
- Keep a spare in case the dummy gets lost.
- Make sure the dummy is smooth and has no cracks in which dirt and germs could become trapped.
- Check the dummy regularly for loose pieces, and throw it away before it becomes old and worn.
- Don't dip the dummy in anything sweet, and don't use a 'dinky feeder' – a type of dummy which you fill with a drink. It could rot your baby's teeth, even before they come through.
- If you are breast-feeding let your baby have some comfort sucks on your breast.
- If you are going out tie or pin the dummy to your baby's clothing to prevent it from getting lost.

at your breast or as he takes his bottle, only to wake with a start the moment you try to put him down.

One of the great advantages of breast-feeding is that you can let your baby suck for comfort if he seems restless. Some babies will go on sucking for hours, which is obviously not practical.

Many babies 'find' their thumbs at about three months of age and suck themselves off to sleep.

Love them or loathe them, dummies or soothers may fulfil your baby's need for sucking. Learning to suck on a dummy may take a little while, however, since the technique is different from that used on bottle or breast. A breast-fed baby may cope better with one of the specially shaped teats that are available.

Using a dummy is unlikely to become a habit before the age of about six months, by which time your baby will have begun to suck on other things such as his hands and toys. If you don't like the look of a dummy, you can quietly 'lose' it before he reaches this age.

Massage The gentle art of massage has had a revival in the last few years. There is nothing quite so effective as a loving touch for soothing a fractious baby. The first time you try it, choose a time when your baby is quiet, but alert, for instance after a feed, bath or when he first wakes up. Start with light, gentle stroking on his chest and fingers and toes. Then gradually work your way over the rest of his body and see how he relaxes and becomes calm and peaceful. A little warmed almond or baby oil will help your hands slide smoothly over his skin, but it is not essential. Make sure the room is comfortably warm, take the phone off the hook and make sure you are uninterrupted for about 10–20 minutes.

Some babies are naturally not very cuddly and do not like being massaged. If you find your baby does not enjoy massage, don't feel you have to persevere.

Swaddling This is another almost infallible way of calming some babies. Newborn babies often wake themselves up just as they are drifting off to sleep by the jerky movements of their arms and legs. They settle better if their movements are restricted. A study of

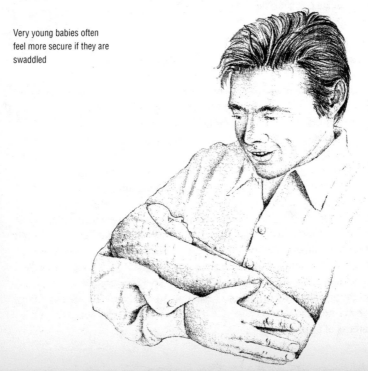

Very young babies often feel more secure if they are swaddled

one-month-old babies shows that swaddling is the most effective way to stop them crying and get them off to sleep. Wrap your baby in a shawl or carrying blanket folded into a triangle, by bringing the top corner diagonally across his body and tucking it under his knees. Now bring the other side across and under his chin, tucking him in so he is a neat little bundle. If he likes to suck his thumb you can wrap him so that he has access to it. After the age of three months your baby will benefit more from having his limbs free than being swaddled.

Another way to make your newborn baby feel cosy and secure is to put him to sleep in a Moses basket, crib or carrycot, or even a well-padded small box or drawer.

Holding Your baby will probably calm down miraculously if you hold him. Many fretful babies respond well to being held firmly facing outwards, so there is slight pressure on their tummy. Alternatively, try holding your baby face downwards across your arm and rocking him briskly. Experiment a little to find the holding position that works best.

If your baby seems to have tummy ache, laying him on his back and exerting firm but gentle pressure against his tummy may calm him.

WHEN THE CRYING DOESN'T STOP

Some babies are naturally more fretful than others. No one quite knows why. Sometimes the cause can be traced to a long, difficult labour, or problems during pregnancy. More often than not a fretful baby just seems to have been born that way.

Such a baby can test your powers of patience to the limit. Your baby's inconsolable wails, combined with your own lack of support, loneliness, exhaustion or inexperience, can try you to the point where you feel you simply cannot cope any longer.

If you have tried the remedies already described and have exhausted any other possibilities, you should seek help from your health visitor or doctor. It can also be useful to talk to other parents who have been through the same agony. Alternatively, contact Crysis (see page 139 for address), an organization that supports and gives practical encouragement to parents of crying babies; or one of the special crying baby clinics that have been set up in some areas of the country for parents of crying babies.

WHAT DO YOUR BABY'S CRIES MEAN?

Sound	*Other clues*
Newborn baby: loud, sudden, urgent.	Roots around, sucks fingers.
Three months onwards: siren-like build-up to loud, demanding scream.	Stretches his body out.
Cries out, grizzles, then moans. If baby is unattended sound becomes a frightened scream.	
Short, shrill screams with pauses in between.	May burp, pass wind or draw up his legs. His stomach may seem hard and swollen.
Whimpers, increasing to loud cry.	Visible soreness or redness in nappy area, baby rubbing ear or drawing up his legs.
Prolonged, high-pitched crying.	
Slight whine and whimper with complaining note, gradually increasing.	Yawns, rubs eyes, seems irritable.
Grizzles irritably.	Chews fists, difficult to comfort. May dribble. Some babies have rashes or loose bowels – though never assume this is just teething; consult your doctor.

Possible cause	What to do
Hunger	Feed baby on demand, even if it's only a short while since his last feed. Increase the number of feeds he has each day: he could be having temporary growth spurt. After four months he may be ready for solids.
Fear of being alone	Go to your baby and pick him up. Carry him around for a while (he may like to be carried in a sling), and talk to him reassuringly. Try some of the remedies on pages 54–7.
Wind	Wind carefully after each feed. Press gently on his tummy. Try giving him a spoonful of warm boiled water or gripe water. Check hole in teat – it could be too large or too small. If you are breast-feeding and your milk is flowing very fast, he may be having to gulp. Try holding him more upright as you feed and taking him off the breast to allow him to get his breath back.
Soreness or discomfort	Check room temperature. When newborn your baby may sleep better if it is 31–2°C (88–90°F). Check back of baby's neck to see if he is sweaty or cold. Adjust clothing and bedding if necessary. Remove obvious causes of pain. If nothing obvious hold him and talk to him reassuringly.
	May indicate pain so consult your doctor.
Overtiredness	Lay him down in a darkened room. Some babies habitually moan for a few minutes before dropping off to sleep. If your baby's jerky movements arouse him, wrap him firmly in his blanket.
Teething	Provide baby with something hard to chew on. Try rubbing an anaesthetic teething gel on his gums. If pain is severe ask doctor if baby could benefit from paracetamol syrup.

Colic

If your baby has a regular crying spell, perhaps in the evenings, during which he screams inconsolably and draws his knees up as though in pain, he could have colic. It is estimated that about three out of ten babies suffer these rhythmic attacks of screaming. Colic usually starts within two weeks of birth and often passes off at around the age of three months – hence the tag 'three-month colic' – although some babies continue to suffer for longer than this.

No one quite knows what causes colic: allergy, heartburn, wind, overfeeding, underfeeding, anxious parents, and an immature baby have all been advanced as possibilities. In other words, the experts don't really know! Very likely it's a combination of some or all of these causes.

As for the cure, many things have been tried and some seem to work for some babies; it seems to be largely a matter of trial and error.

It helps to remember that colic comes to an end eventually, and that it's not your fault. Most babies with colic are in good health, and the colic, wearying though it is for everyone in the family, does no long-term damage.

So what can you do? There is no single, guaranteed remedy: the following are some of the things that have helped some babies.

• If you are breast-feeding keep a careful check on your diet. Some foods seem to cause wind in your baby – oranges, cabbage, onion, coffee, curry are common culprits. You may discover other foods that disagree with your baby, so cut them out of your diet for a while.
• Some babies are upset by dairy foods. If you are bottle-feeding ask your doctor whether it would be a good idea to change to a non-cow's milk formula. If you are breast-feeding cut out butter, cheese, milk, and so on from your diet for a week. Check food labels for 'hidden' dairy products such as whey in biscuits or margarine.
• If you are breast-feeding and your baby wants to suck all the time, and if he is also putting on an excessive amount of weight each week, try cutting down the number of feeds as you could be overfeeding him. It's likely that your baby likes to suck for comfort. Try giving him a dummy or a bottle of plain water.
• Raise the head of your baby's crib or cot by putting a couple of books underneath the legs, to prevent him regurgitating semi-digested feeds into his gullet.
• You need a break occasionally if your baby suffers from colic. Find a sympathetic babysitter and go out with your husband for the evening.
• If nothing you do seems to help, consult your doctor. There are medicines available that help some babies with colic. They should not be administered over long periods, but they can quieten your baby and allow you a little rest.

Tips for parents of a crying baby

- Take your baby for a thorough medical check-up to rule out illness, infection or allergy as a source of crying.
- Remember, your baby will cry less frequently as he gets older and discovers other ways of expressing his needs.
- Keep a diary so you can pinpoint the times your baby is most irritable and maybe assess the reasons.
- Trust your instincts as to how best to care for your baby – they are likely to be right.
- Ignore those who tell you that you will 'spoil your baby' or 'make a rod for your own back' by picking him up every time he cries.
- Don't feel guilty if your baby cries frequently. It's not your fault – some babies are just born that way.
- Some fretfulness before the age of about three or four months is normal.
- Some babies are naturally harder to calm and more easily upset than others.
- You are not alone. Ask your health visitor if there are any support groups or a branch of Crysis in your area that you can contact for advice and information.
- Don't keep your feelings to yourself. If your baby won't stop crying don't hesitate to phone your health visitor for help.
- If you reach the end of your tether, put the baby safely in his cot and go out of the room, to give yourself time to calm down before returning to the fray.

How to cope

If your baby won't stop crying what you need above all – apart from a break in the screams – is a sense of perspective. The following suggestions may help you put your baby's crying in its proper place.

What is he trying to tell me? Your baby's cry may seem like one unbroken grizzle, but if you listen carefully you will notice that he has several different cries, each with its own character. The trick is to learn the clues to your baby's message. It may help to write them down. Note how the cry sounds – is it high-pitched, shrill, sharp, broken?; when it occurs; what you tried and what seemed to help. There are some suggestions in the chart.

- **Keep a diary** Take a tip from the crying baby clinics and note the daily events in baby's life. Keep a record of the times he sleeps, feeds, baths, and so on; and note down anything else that may affect him each day, for example, a change of milk, a visit to the doctor. This will help you to ascertain the times he is always irritable and assess the reasons. He may always cry during the family 'rush hour', for example, when the other children are clamouring for supper, or when you are in a hurry because you have a lot to do.

● **Get to know your baby** If your baby seems to cry frequently it can be difficult to see him as anything other than a demanding little tyrant. By taking special note of the things he seems to like you will begin to see him as the unique person he is. He may love to be cuddled in a warm towel after his bath. He may reward you with a gummy smile when you bounce him on your knee and sing to him. Treasure these moments. Getting to know your baby as a person will help you to understand his special needs.

● **Tune into his moods** If your baby becomes easily fractious you will both get on better if you can avoid forcing him into situations that you know will upset him. For instance, if he's lying in his cot gazing quietly at his mobile, don't choose this time to change his nappy – even though you know it has to be done. Likewise, if he's sitting happily in his chair when visitors call, you can be fairly certain that handing him round from one to another will make him grumpy. You will find that your baby is most responsive when he is in a quiet but alert state. If your baby is the sensitive type, avoid sudden changes and give him plenty of time to become used to anything new. Be sensitive to your baby's signals and bear in mind that you cannot spoil a young baby.

Should I leave him to cry it out?

By and large it's not a good idea to leave a baby to cry. However, there may be occasions when you reach the limit of your patience and it may help to go into another room and calm down. So long as you have made sure that your baby is safe in his cot, he will come to no lasting harm, and you will return to him with renewed energy.

WHEN AN OLDER BABY CRIES

Most of the crying problems we have dealt with are those associated with babies of under three to four months. But what causes older babies to cry and how do you cope? By the time your baby is older you will have come to know him better and learnt the remedies that work best to stop him crying. As your baby grows he will be faced by other situations that might make him cry.

Stranger anxiety
At around the age of seven to eight months your baby, who may previously have been very sociable, suddenly becomes suspicious of people he doesn't know, and cries and clings to you if anyone new approaches him.

What to do Realize that this is an entirely normal phase – about seven out of ten babies suffer stranger anxiety. Stay with your baby to help him feel secure. So long as you are there as his base he will gradually feel less anxious. Let him take his time to become accustomed to a new visitor. Suggest to the visitor that you talk together for a little while before paying any attention to the baby to allow the baby some time to observe the visitor and realize he or she is not threatening. Then the visitor could play a familiar game with the baby, such as peep-bo, or hold out a toy. Alternatively, you can wait for your baby to approach the visitor.

Separation anxiety
Linked to his fear of strangers is a growing reluctance to be separated from you. A baby, who at one time would happily stay with a babysitter, becomes wary and cries when he sees you departing.

What to do Most babies go through this phase and usually grow out of it within a few months, although some babies remain 'shy'. During his 'clingy' period try not to leave him with people he doesn't know well. If you have to leave him never sneak off without saying goodbye, however tempting this may be. Say your farewell and then tell your baby you will be back soon. Even though he doesn't understand what you are saying, he will come to realize, with growing experience, that although you go away you always come back. Give him plenty of love and hugs when you are there. If he has a special comfort object, make sure he always has it with him when you leave.

Frustration
As your baby gets older he'll become more exploratory. If you constantly stop him exploring he will become frustrated, and cry.

What to do Although you must obviously stop your baby doing anything dangerous for his own safety, try to limit the number of times you have to say 'No'. Make sure your house is thoroughly childproof (see pages 128–33). At this age his memory is short and your baby is easily distracted. If he's tormenting the cat, or heading for your toddler's carefully constructed brick house, find something else to attract his attention.

Boredom

As your baby gets older and more active he won't be happy to be left in his cot or chair for long periods. When he gets fed up he will grizzle – you will almost hear the boredom in his voice.

What to do Although you cannot play with your baby every minute of the day, try to spend much of the time with him. The time to catch up on the ironing is when your baby is having his nap, not when he's just woken up and is active. As he gets older his sleep times will be more predictable, enabling you to plan the day better. Arrange various activities, such as a trip to the shops, join a toddler group (they aren't just for toddlers), and visit other mothers with babies. If you have to leave your baby for a while make sure he has interesting things to look at and do (see pages 98–108 for play suggestions). Your baby will be happier if you sit him in a place where he can watch what you are doing.

True or false?

There are lots of myths about babies' crying. Remember you know your baby best, and don't let anyone force you to go against your instincts.
    'You'll spoil your baby if you go to him every time he cries.' FALSE
    'A baby needs to cry to exercise his lungs.' FALSE
    'If you pick up your baby whenever he cries he'll learn bad habits.' FALSE
    'You need to show him who's the boss.' FALSE

ALL ABOUT SLEEP

The idea that a 'good baby' is one who sleeps all the time dies hard. In fact, just like the rest of us, babies vary in their need for sleep. In the early days so long as your baby's needs – for food, drink, warmth and love – are satisfied, you can be sure that she will take the sleep she needs. If your baby needs little sleep in the first few months, your best solution is to adjust your routine so that you have as much rest as you can.

After the age of about three months your baby can be expected to be more settled, and her sleeping patterns will gradually move towards the day-night schedule that we accept as normal. It is during this time that sleeping problems can set in, if you are not careful. There are many ways in which you can encourage your baby to develop an acceptable sleeping pattern, and discourage any bad habits that may become troublesome if allowed to continue.

By the end of her first year your baby will probably be sleeping for over 12 hours, with her main sleep taking place at night, and the rest spread over a couple of naps, morning and afternoon.

At the start

At first your baby will take an average of 16½ hours' sleep each day, and these will be spread fairly randomly around the clock. Even at this early age a day-night rhythm is beginning to emerge, with the time when most babies are likely to be asleep falling between 1 and 3 A.M., and the time they are awake and active between 3 and 8 P.M. – the classic colicky period. Your baby's own in-built biological clock determines the amount of sleep she takes and the time she takes it, and there is little you can do to change this. Some premature babies are extremely sleepy at first; and many full-term babies seem to sleep virtually all the time to begin with; while others never seem to need more than 10 to 12 hours. It is reassuring to know that most babies, given the opportunity, settle down into a more regular routine at some time between three and six months. Just because your baby is a poor sleeper during the early weeks doesn't mean that she will continue to be a night owl for the rest of her life.

Where should my baby sleep?

Your baby will be most comfortable in a crib or carrycot, snugly wrapped in a shawl or cellular blanket to stop the random movements of her arms and legs from waking her as she drifts off to sleep. You may find it convenient to have her next to your bed in your own bedroom at first, so that you can pick her up and feed her when she wakes for a night feed. On the other hand, some parents find their baby's grunts and snuffles too disturbing, and prefer to put her in her own room, or in a corner of another room. Your baby may sleep more soundly if you lay her on a natural sheepskin (not synthetic as the fibres can come loose). In the early weeks lay your baby on her side, so that if she possets up a little of her feed it will drain away from the side of her mouth. By the time she reaches the age of four or five months when she can roll over, you may prefer to let her sleep on her back. Never give a pillow to a baby under a year old as she could suffocate.

Although it is unnecessary to keep absolutely quiet (your baby has to learn to live with the normal household noises), it is a good idea to make a definite distinction between day and night even at this early age. When you put your baby down in the evening, draw the curtains so that the light is dimmed. You may like to put her in a nightie, too, or a special stretch suit or sleeping bag that you keep for night times. Later on she will come to associate her longest sleep time with these night-time rituals. Some recent research has shown that even tiny premature babies, who might be expected not to know the difference between day and night, thrive better and settle more quickly when they are put down to sleep in a special 'night nursery' than when kept in the noisy, bright environment of the daytime special care baby unit.

Your baby will sleep better if she is warm enough. Her room should be around 21°C (70°F). Do not use a paraffin heater in a baby's room – where there is no flue it removes oxygen from the atmosphere. If you have no central heating use a thermostatically controlled electric convector. You can feel if your baby is warm enough by placing your hand on the back of her neck: she should feel just warm, neither hot and sweaty nor cold. Adjust her clothing and bedding accordingly.

Some parents like to let their baby sleep in their own bed in the early months. They claim it makes the baby feel more secure and is convenient for night feeds. Although there is little danger that you will roll over and suffocate your baby (unless you have drunk too much or taken a sleeping tablet), there are one or two points to bear in mind if you decide on a family bed. Many parents, who have started out with the baby in bed, have found that it is an exceptionally hard habit to break once the baby gets older. She becomes so used to having her parents in bed when she falls asleep that she cannot go to sleep without their company. If you have your baby sleeping in your bed, make sure you never leave her in it alone as she could fall off and injure herself. Check your bed for safety, especially if your bed frame has any bars. There are strict safety regulations on the distance between bars on cots, playpens and other items of baby equipment, but they don't apply to adult beds. Once your baby is on the move, she could get her head stuck between the bars, so make sure there is a space of 3–6 cm (1¼–2½ in.) between each one.

Moving to a big cot

Your newborn baby will probably feel more snug and secure in a carrycot or crib. Once she is three or four months old she will start to become too big for it. Now is the time to put her in a big cot. At first many babies feel rather swamped by all the extra space and cry pitifully when you put them down to sleep. Try introducing the cot gradually, by putting her in it only for her daytime sleeps at first. Lining the cot so that it feels more comfy will help, as may putting her to sleep in her carrycot inside the big cot to begin with. Put a few familiar toys and her special comforter, if she has one, inside the cot where she can see them when she goes to sleep.

Sleeping outside

If you have a garden you could put your baby outside in her pram for one or two of her daytime sleeps. Make sure she is not in the direct sun. Put the pram under a tree, or shade her with a parasol or canopy. Cover the pram with a cat net for protection, even if you have no animals of your own.

Settling her into a routine

Between the ages of about three and six months your baby will become more settled. You can help her to develop a regular sleep-wake cycle by introducing a little more routine into her life. In the early months you took your cue from your baby; now, although you should still be guided by her needs, you can help her to feel more secure by starting to follow a flexible schedule. Try to keep her feeds, baths and play periods to particular times of the day, so that she learns to anticipate them. A simple bedtime routine that she knows heralds going to sleep will provide her with regularity and security. It can be planned as follows: playtime, teatime, bathtime, bedtime.

Try not to encourage your baby into the habit of expecting you to rock her, pat her or lie down with her until she drops off. Such habits can often develop into sleeping problems that are hard to remedy. When you take your baby to bed lay her down, tuck her in and perhaps sing a lullaby, then say goodnight and leave her. It will help your baby to feel more secure when you go if she has a special toy or comforter with her.

Cuddlies and comforters

At around the age of seven months or so your baby starts to realize that the objects and people in her life have a permanent existence of their own. This is the time when she begins to become clingy if she sees you go away. She realizes you are separate from her and begins to worry that you won't come back. At around the same age many babies become attached to an object such as a soft toy, a corner of the quilt, or a piece of muslin or blanket. Psychologists call these 'transitional objects', because they substitute the mother when she is not around. They are a stepping stone between dependence and independence. Parents are more likely to call them 'cuddlies' or 'snuggies'.

If your baby develops such an attachment, make sure that her comforter is incorporated into her bedtime routine. Place it in her cot near her so that she can reach for it if she half wakes in the night. It gives her reassurance and comfort, and helps her to accept her separation from you. Don't worry that your baby will become too attached to her comforter – she will grow out of it in her own good time. Only if she appears to prefer her comforter to human company should you consult your health visitor. One last word of advice: your baby is very dependent on her comforter and will be distraught if you lose it. It may be helpful to have two of whatever item she has become attached to, so that if one becomes lost you can quickly replace it.

Be guided by your baby

Some babies have regular sleep patterns and become extremely irritable if they don't have enough sleep. Others are more flexible. You will soon know if your baby is the type who needs a regular 10-hour stretch. How strictly you keep to a sleeping schedule depends very much on your baby's individual personality. A spell of teething, illness, or a visit to relatives can sometimes disrupt her sleeping pattern. If this happens try to return to her normal routine as soon as possible – you'll find tips on how to do this below – otherwise you could be letting yourself in for months of disturbed nights.

Taking your baby away

In the early months your baby is portable. You can tuck her into her basket or carrycot and take her with you wherever you go. However, after the age of eight months your baby will become more settled if you keep to a recognizable bedtime routine. If you go out in the evening, it is best to settle her and leave her with a reliable babysitter rather than take her with you. You will benefit from the break too.

When you have to take your baby with you, for instance when you go away to stay with relatives or friends, or on holiday, try to follow her normal bedtime schedule as closely as possible. Take your own sheets and bedding, her favourite toys, and special comforter if she has one. Aim to give her her bath at the same time as she usually has it at home, and tuck her in and say goodnight as you normally would. Avoid undue excitement at bedtime: ask relatives or friends to say their goodnights before you take her for her bath, and spend a little time calming her so that she is relaxed and ready to sleep.

Sleep problems

During the first few months of your baby's life any problems with sleeping are more likely to be yours (not enough of it!) than hers. Accept that your baby will gradually become more settled and try to catch up on your sleep during the day, or by snatching an occasional early night.

Later on your baby becomes able to resist sleep, even though you know she must be tired. Some babies develop rituals that can prove exceptionally hard to break. Parents who have developed the habit of rubbing, patting, rocking or feeding the baby until she sleeps, can be at a loss to know how to cope when their baby wakes several times a night and refuses to go back to sleep without this attention.

If this happens to you, bear in mind that *it will get better*. Giving your baby medication is rarely the answer. You need to help your baby break the habit of associating rubbing, patting, feeding or whatever with going to sleep, and teach her to fall asleep on her own. This means that you will have to be prepared to cope with some crying for a few nights. It will be easier on you and your baby if you change her pattern gradually and progressively. A method that has been successfully used in sleep clinics is outlined in the box below.

It's best to start any new sleeping regimes at a weekend or on holiday when it won't matter so much if you miss out on some sleep. It may be a good idea for you and your husband to take turns to attend to the baby. If you always breast-feed your baby to sleep, letting her father go to see her may well dispel the habit more quickly, as she will have learnt to associate you with being fed.

Helping your baby to fall asleep alone

Put your baby down and tuck her in. Say goodnight and leave. If she cries wait 15 minutes. Then if she is still crying hard, go in and talk to her gently and reassuringly to let her know you are still there.

Don't pick her up or rock, pat, stroke or feed her however tempted you might be to do so – you will only extend the time it takes to settle her in alone.

After a few minutes leave her again. Carry on with this process until she eventually falls asleep.

Be prepared to persevere – it takes a while for her to unlearn her previous habits.

If your baby's bedtime is unacceptably late, once the new pattern is established you can gradually bring forward her bedtime by half an hour a week.

Use the method outlined above for encouraging your baby to take her daytime naps. Persevere until she has become used to going to sleep on her own. The same process can also be used if, for any reason, your baby has deviated from her usual sleep pattern. Continue with it until she returns to her normal routine.

This method really does work, as many parents can testify. The secret is to make any change gradual and progressive – and to persevere.

Night waking

Some night waking is to be expected in a baby under a year old. We all surface momentarily several times a night, but we usually drop off to sleep again, and unless something reminds us we don't even remember in the morning. If you hear your baby stir and you are no longer giving night feeds, leave her for a few minutes to settle. If she carries on crying, check to see what is wrong, make sure she is warm enough, and keep attention low key and to the minimum. A night light installed in her room may help to comfort her if she wakes. The tips on soothing your baby (see pages 54–7) will help you to cope if your baby cries when she wakes.

Early morning waking

Some babies develop the habit of waking at five or six in the morning and refusing to settle. They often have a nap early in the morning, because their early rising hour has made them quickly sleepy. The way to overcome the problem is to make getting-up time and nap time

gradually later. For instance, if she regularly wakes at 5 A.M. and has a
nap at 9.30 A.M., on the first day leave her in her cot until 5.15 A.M.
and don't put her down for her nap until 10 A.M. Give her a few days to
adjust to this new pattern, then move both getting-up time and nap
time forward by another 15 minutes. Repeat this until your baby starts
sleeping to a more acceptable hour – say 7 A.M. You will probably find
that, after the first few days, she will begin to drop off to sleep again in
the morning for another couple of hours.

However, some babies are by nature 'larks' and others are 'owls', just
like the rest of us. If your baby is a natural early riser, you can try to

---

Helping your baby to sleep

Tips for help with newborn babies
- In the first couple of months your baby may feel more secure and snug if
  you wrap her or swaddle her (see chapter on crying, pages 56–7).
- From the start try to make a definite distinction between day and night.
  When you put your baby down to sleep in the evening draw the curtains
  and dress her in nightclothes.
- Make sure your baby's room is warm enough. In the winter you may like
  to warm her cot with an electric blanket or hot-water bottle, which
  should be removed before laying your baby down to sleep. In the summer
  you may need to open a window if it is very hot and cover her with very
  little bedding.
- Use any of the tips listed in the chapter on crying (see pages 54–7) to
  help your baby relax and fall asleep.

Tips for help with babies aged 6 months–1 year
- Keep bedtime calm and happy.
- Work out a bedtime routine and, as far as possible, adhere to it.
- Encourage your baby to develop ways of comforting herself, for example
  with a comforter.
- Don't take your baby out with you in the evenings.
- If your baby wakes up in the night, give her time to settle again. Don't
  automatically pick her up.
- If your baby cries out suddenly, comfort her perhaps by patting her back
  and talking softly to her, but avoid picking her up.
- Avoid developing rituals such as rubbing, patting, rocking or feeding as
  methods of getting your baby to sleep.
- Make sure your baby's room is warm enough.
- If your baby is easily disturbed by noise, line the curtains at her bedroom
  window and put thick carpet on the floor to muffle sounds.
- Install a low night light in the room which may comfort your baby and
  help her to settle.

delay her getting-up time by keeping her room dark – hang thick lined curtains at the window – and waiting before you go to her, in order to give her the chance to drift off to sleep again. You may also be able to enjoy a few minutes' extra sleep for yourself by making sure she has a few toys in her cot to occupy her. You may simply have to accept that she is an early riser and look forward to the day when she is old enough to get up by herself.

Your baby's sleep in the first year

Age	Sleep time
One week	16½ hours: about eight hours at night and the rest spread out throughout the day.
One month	15½ hours: about nine hours at night and three naps of a couple of hours or so each during the day.
Three months	15 hours: about 10 hours at night and a couple of long naps and one short one during the day.
Six months	14½ hours: about 11 hours at night and a couple of long daytime naps, morning and afternoon.
Nine months	14 hours: about 11 hours at night and one short and one long daytime nap.
One year	13¾ hours: about 11 hours at night and two short daytime naps, morning and afternoon.

Although the above is a typical pattern, remember that your baby is a unique individual and may take more or less sleep than this. Bear in mind that your baby, especially in the early months, is not being deliberately naughty if she doesn't sleep much.

Going to sleep late

If your baby never goes to sleep until late in the evening, it could be that her last daytime nap is scheduled too late in the day. If she regularly has a nap from 4 P.M. to 6 P.M. it is unreasonable to expect her to go to bed again at 7 P.M. and you need to move her afternoon nap to an earlier time. Again, the best way to do this is to move the nap time gradually back, by a quarter of an hour every couple of days or so, while, at the same time, bringing her bedtime forward by the corresponding period. If she has a morning nap as well, you may also need to adjust the time of this.

Part IV

LEARNING ABOUT THE WORLD

YOUR BABY'S DEVELOPMENT

During the first year your baby grows from a tiny newborn, whose only language is crying and who relies on you to do everything for him, to a lively enquiring little child, who is beginning to walk and talk. You will be astonished at the rate of his progress. Never again will he develop so quickly.

Of all baby animals the human baby is the most 'unfinished' at birth – on account of his large brain! But even though your baby seems capable of little more than sucking, crying, excreting and sleeping, this is far from the whole story.

In fact, your newborn baby is possessed of some amazing abilities, which literally programme him for learning. You can help by being tuned into his changing needs, so that you can provide the opportunities he needs to develop new skills and abilities.

Did you know that:

- Your baby recognizes your face within hours of birth?
- Your newborn baby recognizes his own native language?
- Your baby knows your voice at birth and will turn to try to locate the source of a sound?
- Your newborn baby responds to a story he heard in the womb?
- Your baby distinguishes your smell from that of other mothers within a couple of days of birth?
- Your baby prefers sweet tastes at just a day old?
- Your baby focuses up to distances of 150 cm (5 ft.), although he sees clearest at about 20 cm (8 in.) – about the distance you are from him as you care for him?

Not so long ago it was believed that a baby's mind was a blank sheet at birth, but today it is realized that a baby's senses are all in good working order, and his intellectual and perceptual apparatus is prepared for development.

One of the most fascinating and rewarding aspects of being a parent is watching this little human being grow and develop. All babies go through the same stages of development. But how fast your baby moves from one stage to the next depends on a number of things – his genes, his experiences inside the womb and in the world, how healthy he is, his place in the family, and so on. There is little you can do to hurry your baby's development, as he is born with his own biological clock that determines its progress. No amount of placing your baby on his tummy will force him to crawl until he is ready. It helps to bear this in mind whenever you feel tempted to measure your baby's development against that of another child who is progressing faster.

What you can do is provide plenty of opportunities for your baby, so that when he is mature enough to acquire a particular skill he is able to do so. For example, once he starts pulling himself up against the furniture, make sure he has plenty of sturdy, stable surfaces close enough together to cruise around. You will find tips on the sorts of activities to provide him with in the section on play (see page 98).

Your baby will progress spasmodically from one milestone to the next. Once he has acquired a new skill or ability he needs time to

---

Isn't he doing well?

Points to remember:

- Your baby's development takes place in a set order, which is the same for every baby, but how fast he develops depends on his own in-built time clock.
- Your baby develops from head to toe. He cannot crawl until he can hold up his head. He cannot walk until he can sit and crawl.
- Your baby develops from the middle outwards. He learns to control his upper arms and legs earlier than his lower arms, legs, hands and feet.
- Your baby's movements gradually become more refined. At first he makes large, jerky movements using his whole body and later on he develops more delicate control of his small muscles, until by the end of his first year he can pick up a crumb between finger and thumb.
- Your baby develops at an uneven rate. Once he has mastered a new ability his progress will halt for a while before he takes another bound forward.
- Your baby acquires each new skill and activity when he is ready. Unless you keep him locked in a dark room deprived of all stimulus your baby will develop – because he's programmed to do so.
- Be sure to take your baby for all his developmental check-ups to ensure that he is progressing as he should.
- Resist the temptation to compare your baby with others of the same age – he is a unique individual.

practise and perfect it before moving on to the next stage. He may sometimes seem to 'forget' a skill that he previously mastered. He hasn't really forgotten it – he is simply concentrating on his next achievement.

Even though your baby follows a pre-set sequence of development he may miss out on a stage or evolve his own peculiar way of doing something. For instance, some babies miss out on the crawling stage and move straight on to walking. Others move from one place to another by shuffling on their bottoms or by doing a strange, crab-like half walk, half crawl.

From time to time there may be interruptions or delays in your baby's progress. For example, if he is ill, or if he experiences some other upset such as a house move, he may revert to an earlier stage of behaviour. A baby who was happy being spoon-fed may temporarily want breast- or bottle-feeding. If this occurs, comply for a while and he will soon be back to normal.

If your baby was born early you can expect him to be a little later than average in reaching the various milestones up to the age of one or two.

CONTROL OF BODY AND MOVEMENTS

At birth most of your baby's movements are reflex (automatic reactions over which he has no control). Gradually, over the course of the next few months, many of these instinctive movements are replaced by deliberate ones.

Reflexes		
● Rooting reflex	● Grasp reflex	● Walking reflex
● Blink reflex	● Startle reflex (Moro)	● Stepping reflex

In order to make a deliberate action your baby has to learn to associate what he does with what happens – that is, cause and effect. For instance, at first when he sucks at the breast or bottle his sucking is purely instinctive. Gradually, over the next few weeks, he learns that when he sucks milk flows, and the instinctive sucking reflex is replaced by deliberate sucking actions.

Controlling the head

Your newborn baby cannot control his head because his neck muscles
are weak. If you hold him forward his head will droop.

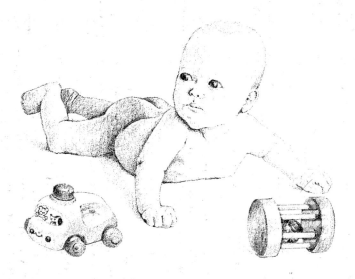

At six weeks your baby's neck has become stronger. He can raise his
head in line with his body for a moment or so.
At three months he can lift his head in line with his body and hold it
there for some time. If you put him on his front he will raise his head
and upper chest and peer around, using his forearms for support. If he
sleeps on his front you may see him peering over the edge of his carrycot
or crib when he wakes up.
By six months he has full control of his head. He bears the weight of his
body on his hands to raise himself up. If he is lying on his back he lifts
his head to peer at his toes – a source of endless fascination!

Learning to crawl

If you lay your newborn baby on his tummy he draws his knees up under
his tummy and lies with his head to one side.

By six weeks he has uncurled and lies with his legs stretched out. He can raise his head and keep it upright before it wobbles down again.
At three months he lies with his legs completely stretched. He presses on his hands to push up his chin and shoulders.
At four months he lifts his chest and legs off the floor as though he is a swimmer.
By five months he leans on his forearms and confidently looks around.

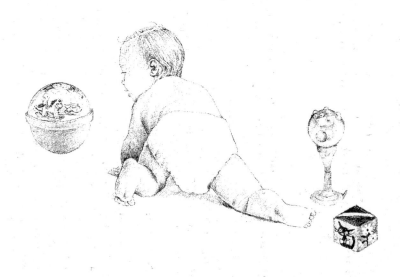

By six months he can support the top of his body and, with arms outstretched, he uses his hands to support himself. He may adopt a crawling position and rock backwards and forwards.
At seven months he can support himself on one hand alone.
At eight months he starts to creep by pressing down with his hands and kicking with his legs . . . but to his – and your – surprise he moves backwards!
By nine months he can propel himself forwards but his legs still trail behind him.
At 11 months he is fully co-ordinated and will crawl confidently around the room. Make sure it's child proof!

Learning to sit up

Your newborn baby slumps forwards if you hold him in a sitting position.

At one month his back is still rounded, but he lifts his head for a moment or so if you hold him sitting up.

At three months he will hold his head up, although it is still inclined to droop forward.

At four months his lower back is still rounded but his head is erect. It will still wobble if his body sways.

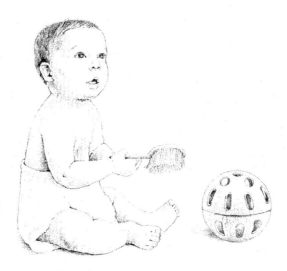

At five months he still needs your support, but his head is now steady and his back is straight.

At six months he lifts his head for you to pull him up. He sits upright supported in his pram or highchair.

At seven months he can sit up alone, although he still has to steady himself with his hands, and he is inclined to wobble over.

At eight months he can sit unaided, but he is still a little wobbly.

At nine months he is sitting well and can maintain his position for 10 minutes. He leans forward confidently to pick things up without losing his balance.

Standing and walking

Your newborn baby walks across the table when he is held – but it's only a reflex.

At two months he holds up his head for a moment or so if you hold him in a standing position.

At six months he loves to use his legs to bounce on your lap when you hold him upright.

At seven months he hops and dances from one foot to the other.

At nine months he pulls himself up against the furniture and stands. If

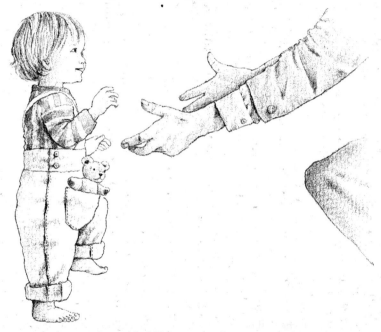

you take his weight and hold him in a walking position he will put one foot in front of the other, but he can't yet balance and you must be sure to support him.

At 10 or 11 months he begins to walk holding on to the furniture. If you hold his hands he will walk forwards.

At around about a year he walks forward with you holding on to one of his hands.

He takes off on his own! This may be at any time from nine to 18 months.

Manipulation

At birth your baby's hands are tightly closed. If you place anything in his hand or stroke his palm the grasp reflex causes him to grip it tightly or make a fist.

At two months his hands are no longer closed and he may grasp things momentarily.

At three months he can hold a rattle, but he doesn't yet know how to reach out for things – you have to place them in his hand. He is fascinated by his hands and will watch them in front of his face.

At four months he loves to play with his hands. He clasps and unclasps them, and sucks them, just for fun.

At five months he grasps objects, although his hold is still a little insecure.

At six months he curls fingers and thumb around an object, such as a block or small ball, and twists it so he can examine it. He will pass an object from hand to hand and love banging it on the floor.

At seven months he holds an object in each hand – but he still has trouble letting go. Beware of your hair!

At eight months he grips a cube with his thumb opposite his fingers, using a pincer-like grasp.

At nine months his thumb and finger grip is delicate enough to pick up

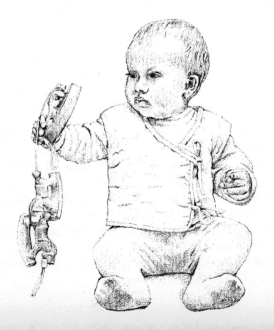

a small object such as a pea. He starts to poke with his forefinger – and meal times become a messy business.

By 10 months he can handle two objects at once, and he is learning to let go. Help him release his grip by holding your hand out flat when he puts something on it.

At a year he can feed himself and hold a crayon. He knows how to let go and he will delight in practising this new-found skill by handing you toys and even bits of his dinner!

Helping your baby to develop physically

- Be guided by your baby's developing skills and abilities. At first you will have to support his head carefully. As his neck becomes stronger you will be able to carry him upright without constantly holding his head.
- Play games that involve gently pulling him up and lowering him again.
- Support him with cushions where he can see what's going on. Experiment with different types of baby chair that give him varying degrees of support and a different view of the world.
- Don't always put your baby down in the same position. Varying his position and posture helps develop different muscles and gives him different views. Sometimes he will like to lie and gaze at the mobile you have hung above his pram. At other times he will like to raise himself on his arms and peer over the side of his carrycot.
- Once he starts to rock on all fours you can encourage him to crawl by placing toys just out of his reach, to attract him forward.
- Babies learn by copying. Once he is on all fours, let him see you crawling.
- Help him exercise his legs. Give him things to kick against: your hands or body as he is lying on your lap; soft blocks or a pillow filled with crinkly paper placed at the bottom of his crib or cot.
- As he gets older let him bounce on your lap and on the floor. A baby bouncer is a good investment at this stage.
- To help your baby stand leave his socks off, so that he can grip with his toes.
- Once he starts to shuffle along, move furniture close together to enable him to cruise around it.
- Don't force your baby to do things before he is ready or he will lose confidence and become discouraged.

PHYSICAL GROWTH AND WEIGHT GAIN

Babies come in all shapes and sizes. If you or your husband are slight and wiry, your child is likely to take after you. Your baby's growth is determined by her genes, her general health and the diet you give her. There is some evidence that babies whose parents are overweight grow faster in the first year, although whether this is caused by an inherited tendency to be large, or by diet, is as yet uncertain. Big babies tend to gain weight faster than small ones. But if your baby was small as a result of being premature or because of intrauterine growth retardation (failure to grow properly in the womb) she will probably catch up later.

Your baby will not gain weight evenly, but is likely to grow in fits and starts. If she has been ill, teething or off her food, her progress may slow down for a while, but she will make up for such temporary lulls by having a growth spurt. Generally, she will grow faster in the spring and summer and slower in the autumn and winter.

GROWTH CHARTS

Heights and weights are all averages, and boys are slightly larger and taller than girls.

HEIGHT

Age	Boys	Girls
Newborn	50.5 cm (20 in.)	49.5 cm (19¾ in.)
Three months	60.5 cm (24 in.)	59.5 cm (23¾ in.)
Six months	66.5 cm (26½ in.)	65.5 cm (26 in.)
Nine months	71 cm (28½ in.)	70 cm (28 in.)
One year	75 cm (30 in.)	74 cm (29½ in.)

WEIGHT

Age	Boys	Girls
Newborn	3.4 kg (7 lb. 7 oz.)	3.3 kg (7 lb. 5 oz.)
Three months	5.5 kg (12 lb. 2 oz.)	5.4 kg (12 lb.)
Six months	7.5 kg (16 lb. 8 oz.)	7.25 kg (16 lb.)
Nine months	9 kg (19 lb. 12 oz.)	8.7 kg (19 lb.)
One year	10.2 kg (22 lb. 8 oz.)	10 kg (22 lb.)

There is a wide variation in 'normal' height and weight, and so long as your baby is putting on weight and gaining height in relation to her own starting point, she is likely to be doing well. If she stops growing for some unexplained reason (i.e. she hasn't been ill, etc.) consult your health visitor or doctor.

Changing proportions

Your baby's brain is large, which accounts for her big, wobbly head. By contrast, her body is small and undeveloped. Over the course of the first year her head and body become more evenly proportioned. Her body is chubby and she has a rounded belly. Her legs are bowed, giving her a waddling gait, and her feet are podgy and flat.

How your baby perceives the world

Your baby's senses are all in good working order at birth. You can help to introduce him to the world around him if you imagine how it must appear to him. The following pages will give you some idea of how your baby experiences the world.

Seeing

Your newborn baby can see surprisingly well. Even at a day old he can distinguish the edges of vertical stripes at a distance of 23–30 cm (9–12 in.). He can see in three dimensions and focus on objects about 20 cm (8 in.) away from his face. This ability seems related to his capacity for being sociable – 20 cm (8 in.) is about the distance between him and the face of the person who is feeding him or changing his nappy.

Your baby is attracted to bold geometric shapes, with strong contrasts. He is also captured by movement and will fix his eyes on a moving object for a short time.

Above all, he is excited by the human face, which has all the elements that hold a baby's attention. It has a clear outline, it is constantly moving, and there is plenty of contrast between the eyes and hair and the rest of the face.

According to the experts, babies see the world not in terms of shape and form as we do, but in terms of prominent features that are spread across the field of sight. It is thought that the reason for this is to enable them to place an object in its context before examining it in detail.

As for colour, your baby prefers medium tones like mid-yellow, green or pink, rather than bright blues, orange, red or more subtle shades such as grey, fawn or beige. He likes lots of strong contrasts, black and white checkerboard patterns, circles, dots and squares at least 8 cm (3 in.) tall.

When your baby is just a few hours old he will track a moving object with both eyes. He has to adjust his vision more than adults do, as his eyes have to move through a wider angle to get an object back into the centre of his field of vision, once he's lost sight of it.

You can use these observations to help your baby. When you show him something hold him about 20 cm (8 in.) from it, and give him plenty of time to fix his gaze on it and explore it with his eyes. Hold a rattle or toy the same distance away from him, slowly move it across his field of vision and watch him follow it with his eyes. Put interesting pictures around his cot, and suspend a mobile above it made up of geometric shapes such as bold circles in black and white.

Until your baby is about eight to 10 weeks old he may squint, because at first he has difficulty in getting both eyes to work together. At around this age he begins to co-ordinate his eyes. If he continues to squint after the age of three months, see your doctor, so that he or she can monitor any imbalance of his eye muscles and correct them if necessary.

From three months old your baby is beginning to become more interested in the fine detail of the things he sees. Throughout the whole of his first year he prefers to look at round shapes and circular patterns, or anything that is face-shaped. He will minutely examine the features of your face, and those of other members of the family.

By the time your baby is a year old his vision is as good as it will ever be. Now all that remains is for him to learn to interpret what he sees.

KEEPING A CHECK ON YOUR BABY'S PROGRESS

Your baby's development will be checked at regular intervals by your doctor and health visitor, so that any problems or delays in her development can be picked up at an early stage.

DEVELOPMENTAL CHECK-UPS

Check	What the doctor is looking for
Six weeks	Any minor problems that may have been overlooked during earlier checks in hospital. Developing muscle tone: how well your baby holds her head up. Weight gain: your baby will now be gaining weight regularly at about a rate of 170–227 gm (6–8 oz.) a week. Focusing: the doctor may move a toy in front of her face to watch how she follows it with her eyes. Newborn reflexes.
Six to eight months	Physical development: rolling, sitting, head lift, strength of legs. If the doctor or health visitor is unable to record these abilities from observation, you will be asked to list what your baby can do. Use of hands: the doctor may hand your baby a block to see how she manipulates it. Eyesight: check to ensure she is not squinting. Hearing: a test may be carried out at your home, separately from the developmental check. Intellectual and social skills: observation of how your baby responds to you, how she tries to copy your speech, sound and movements.
10 months to a year (not all doctors carry out a check at this age)	Physical development: whether she takes her full weight on her feet and pulls herself up on furniture. Manipulative skills: she may be given blocks to play with to test these skills. Intellectual and social skills: your baby may be asked to wave goodbye or clap her hands. The doctor will listen to the sounds she makes, and may test her understanding by talking to her or showing her pictures in a book.

Special developmental checks are held either at your doctor's surgery or the local child health clinic, run by your District Health Authority, in which case the check may be performed by a community paediatrician and the health visitor. The timing of the check-ups varies slightly from one area to another, but generally your baby's progress is checked at six weeks, six to eight months, and at 10 months to one year.

A thorough check is made for progress in four areas of your baby's development:

- Large body movements – the development of control over head and limbs, and the progress of such skills as crawling, sitting, walking, and so on.
- Fine body movements – co-ordination of hand and eye movements, ability to pick up small objects, focus eyes, etc.
- Hearing and language – tests for hearing and understanding language.
- Social development – the way your baby interacts with you and with others around her.

SOCIAL DEVELOPMENT

Your baby is a social creature. Every aspect of his development is geared to this fact, so it is hard to separate his progress as a social being from his progress in understanding and other areas of development.

Newborn Your baby already recognizes your face and the sound of your voice. He tries to follow you with his eyes.

One month He watches you intently as you talk and tries to copy you. He stops crying when you lift him up. Some time between now and six weeks he gives his first social smile that you know is just for you.

Three months He welcomes you with a smile when you draw near his pram or cot. He hates being left alone and cries for company. He recognizes members of his family and other people he sees regularly. He starts to be a little wary of strangers and may cry if a strange person approaches him.

Four months He becomes excited when he sees you preparing to feed or bath him. He lifts his arms for you to pick him up. He enjoys 'talking' to you. He laughs and giggles with delight when you play with him.

Six months By now he is really sociable. He pulls your hair and pats your face. He likes to look at himself in the mirror, although he's not quite sure who it is!

Eight months He knows his name. He understands when you say 'No'. He actively tries to grab your attention by shouting, and copies your speech, sound and gestures.

Nine months He's starting to get a mind of his own. He may protest when you dress him, or try to crawl off when you put on his nappy. If he doesn't like wearing a hat he pulls it off and hurls it to the ground. He's quite shy of strangers, but will watch from the safety of your lap and, if left to himself, may eventually approach the stranger. He obeys simple instructions and understands quite a few simple words and phrases.

One year He understands about 20 words. He loves to make you laugh and repeats anything that you find amusing. He likes to look at picture books and point to objects. He helps you dress him by holding out an arm or leg. He may say one or two simple words.

INTELLECTUAL DEVELOPMENT

At some time between the age of nine and 18 months your baby utters her first 'real' word. It's a thrilling moment, but in fact she has been working up to that first recognizable word ever since she was born; and possibly even before. Babies just a few hours old have been shown on film moving in synchrony with someone talking to them; using body language to regulate the flow of conversation in just the same way as two adults talking to each other.

At one time psychologists believed that a baby entered the world in a state of 'buzzing, booming confusion'. It is now realized that, even though a baby is largely physically helpless, her brain is all set to learn. She is literally programmed to acquire and process all the information that is coming in through her senses.

The development of speech is closely tied to your baby's growth of understanding. In order to understand and make sense of the world, your baby has to be able to pay attention, to perceive and to remember. Her memory enables her to appreciate that the objects around her – her

bottle, her favourite teddy, the family pet – which at first seem to
appear and disappear magically in fact have a separate, permanent
existence of their own. With this realization comes the learning that
you give names to these objects. As you hand her that cuddly thing,
you say, 'Here's your teddy,' and gradually your baby learns to associate
the word you use with this furry object she likes to stroke. These two
insights are important parts of learning to talk. After all, without the
recognition that things have names, there can be no communication.
And unless she realizes that things continue to exist even though she
can't see them, there is little point in naming them or in talking about
them. You can help your baby by showing an interest in her and her
activities, and introducing her to the fascination of language.

At first your baby is busy amassing information about the world
around her through her senses. Above all she is fascinated by people
and longs to communicate. Include her in your family activities right
from the start. Prop her up where she can see you going about your daily
tasks.

Your baby's mind collects and stores every scrap of information that
comes in through her senses. Even a tiny baby has a rudimentary
memory. If you present your baby with a new experience she pays close
attention to it. Try shaking a rattle she hasn't seen before, or showing
her a new mobile, and watch how she gazes intently at it, taking in
every aspect of its shape and form. After a while she loses interest in it
and starts to pay attention again only when you present her with
something new. This ability to 'turn off' sensations and experiences
that have become stale and familiar enables her to learn astonishingly
quickly. By filing away information in her memory where she can call
on it for future reference, she is able to concentrate on what is new, so
building up a store of knowledge about the world around her with
amazing speed.

Like all the best filing systems, your baby's memory is infinitely
adaptable. Say you hold out a wooden block to her. She shapes her
hand in order to take it from you. Then next day you hand her a ball.
This time she has to alter the shape of her grasp. If she tries to handle it
in the way she did for the block she will drop it. It takes a while before
she gets it right, but eventually she succeeds in holding this fascinating
new object. You'll see her twist and turn it, transfer it from hand to
hand and explore it with her mouth, as she takes in all its properties.
Once she has fully explored it, she logs all the new information away

in her mental filing cabinet. In this way your baby becomes extraordinarily competent in a whole range of tasks.

You can help her build up her knowledge of the world by providing her with plenty of varied experiences. Once you can see she is bored with the mobile that is hanging over her cot, put up a new one. When she is familiar with the pictures you have stuck on her wall, change them. Make sure she doesn't have the same toys to play with all the time. You'll find hints on the type of games and toys she will like on pages 98–108.

It's still there!

At first your baby's memory is only primitive. By four months she recognizes you and her father and any other members of the family she sees regularly. She knows when it is time for her feed or bath and reacts eagerly when she sees you making the familiar preparations. But as yet her memory is restricted. She can't think about things when they are not there. Out of sight is out of mind, and once an object is no longer physically present, it is as though it doesn't exist. If she drops a toy she is playing with, it has gone and she won't bother to search for it.

As your baby gains increasing control over her limbs and movements she becomes more actively exploratory and so gains more knowledge, until one day at around the age of nine months it dawns on her that even though she cannot see an object it is still there. This realization marks a big step forward in her development. After all, without the knowledge that objects have an existence of their own, there is nothing to talk about. Your baby will try out this new-found recognition by hurling toys to the floor for you, or anyone who is willing, to retrieve. This is the age too when she delights in games of hide-and-seek, such as peep-bo. Now she knows that things exist, she has a reason to learn their names; and this knowledge forms the basis of conversation.

Even though her memory is still short it begins now to include the past. Now if you go away she begins to miss you, and this is the reason so many babies enter a clingy phase around this age.

Cause and effect

A vital part of your baby's growing understanding is an awareness of cause and effect. Conversation is, after all, a two-way process: if I say one thing you will react.

Right from the start your baby is interested in 'happenings'. It used to be thought that a baby acquired a knowledge of cause and effect only through a long process of trial and error. However, recent research has shown that even babies as young as three months have some rudimentary understanding of cause and effect, e.g. hunger crying and being given food.

Gradually as your baby gains more control over her movements she starts to put this awareness into practice. For example, if you hang a number of objects across her cot, at first she swipes one accidentally. As she watches it swing and rattle she may bash it again. Gradually she begins to realize that it is her own action that has caused this to happen.

By the time she is between about eight months to a year old she has become very deliberate in her actions. The development of her memory makes it possible for her to predict that if she does a particular thing, something else will happen.

STAGES IN LEARNING TO TALK

Although your new baby can't talk, she can make herself understood. Unpromising as they seem, all those cries, gurgles, coos and other noises she makes pave the way for the day when she utters her first real word. She's practising using her vocal cords but, equally important, she's learning that the noises she makes have an effect. She's hungry. She cries. As if by magic you come and feed her. She soils her nappy. She grizzles miserably. Miraculously you come and make her clean and dry. Your baby is learning important lessons from these experiences – sounds have meaning; what she does has an effect on those around her.

As she gets older your baby's repertoire of responses grows. One day at around four months she lets out a wild, joyful chuckle. You are delighted and show it. She laughs again. It's so infectious, you laugh back – and so it goes on, back and forth, just like a conversation.

Even at birth your baby is fully attuned to the sound of the human voice. She'll turn to the sound of your voice to try to see where it's coming from. Even at birth your baby has the ability to co-ordinate sensations coming from two different senses – sound and vision. She automatically knows that a sound must come from someone or something she can see. It's thought that it's this ability that enables your baby to recognize you as her mother when she is merely hours old. Recent research has also shown that babies are attuned to their own native language. It's likely that your baby picks up patterns of speech and stress while in the womb that enable her to recognize her own language when she is born.

In order to talk your baby has to acquire three vital skills:

- She has to make sounds that make sense to other people.
- She has to understand what others are saying to her.
- She has to realize that conversation is a two-way affair and learn to take turns.

As you can see these three skills are closely linked to her growing understanding.

In order to speak your baby has to master over 40 different speech sounds. It's thought that when your baby 'babbles' she is actually practising the sounds she will later use in speech, without having to make sure that they mean something. Some sounds, such as 'a', are mastered early on. Others, such as 's', 'f', 'h', 'r', 'th', take much longer to learn, and she may still be mispronouncing words by the time she starts school.

Long before she says her first word she understands what you say to her. She will probably be able to understand about 20 words even though she can't yet say any. For instance, if you ask her 'Where's daddy?' she may look towards the door, as though expecting him to come in. If you tell her to point to the light, she may well obey your instruction even though it will be many months before she says the word 'light'. If you have ever been to a foreign country, you will realize that this ability to recognize what is said before you can actually speak the language yourself is one that persists throughout life.

Your baby's first word will probably be a name such as 'mama', or 'dada', the name of a familiar toy such as the plastic duck that floats in her bath, 'du', or family pets such as 'ca' (cat) or 'do' (dog). At this stage she makes words work hard for her. One sound such as 'da' can have many meanings. It can mean 'that', 'duck', 'dog', 'thank you'.

Learning to talk – how your baby progresses

Newborn Your baby cannot use language, but she manages to make her needs known. You will find that you automatically know the right way to talk to your baby. You will instinctively modulate the tone, pitch and pace of your speech when talking to her. As well as crying your baby makes other recognizable sounds: a gurgle of contentment, a peaceful cooing. She moves her arms and legs in synchrony as you speak to her. She knows the sound of your voice.

Six weeks Your baby is beginning to take turns – a vital part of conversation. When you talk to her she becomes quiet and listens intently. When you stop she gurgles back at you, then waits for you to say something else.

Three months Now your baby is becoming more vocal. When she's happy she softly coos to herself. You will soon find yourself cooing back. In this way your baby learns that conversation is two-way. Her repertoire of sounds increases. She positively squeals with pleasure when you play a game she likes. She is beginning to make 'proper' sounds too: she will start with consonants, such as 'p', 'b', 'm', 'k' and 'g', and vowels, such as 'a', 'o' or 'e'. As she gains control of her muscles she tries to copy you. Try blowing a raspberry and watch her imitate it.

Five to seven months Psychologists call this period the time of 'vocal play', when your baby repeats the same sounds over and over again for the sheer fun of it. She loves to imitate the sounds you make. At seven months the sounds she makes become more like those of adult speech. She uses her lips and tongue to say 'ba' and 'da'.

Eight to 12 months During this time, or earlier, your baby begins to 'babble': to string sounds together like 'ba-ba-ba', 'da-da-da'. She pauses and puts expression into her voice just as if she is having a real conversation. The more you respond to her the more she babbles. She calls for your attention and shows she understands a lot of what you are saying. If you ask her to 'Wave bye-bye' or 'Clap hands' she willingly obliges, and delights in showing off her new skills to everyone.

As understanding dawns she begins to use the noises she makes to produce some sort of action. She drops her rattle and orders you to pick it up – even though she's not using words, the meaning is unmistakable! She calls to you to get her food. She is on the brink of real speech.

Around this time she begins to use 'scribble talk', or 'jargon'. She joins up syllables, using the rising and falling intonation of real speech, in such a way that you find yourself straining to catch what she is saying!

Finally, at some time around now she may say her first real word. It will be a while before other people realize what your baby is saying, but you and the other members of the family will be in no doubt what she is trying to communicate. From now on there'll be no stopping her.

How to help your baby learn to talk

- Spend some time with her every day free of other distractions such as television, radio, other children, and so on.
- Look at her when you talk to her so she can copy you.
- Talk about the familiar things in her world – feeding, dressing, going out, her toys, members of her family, pets. To your baby all these things are fascinating, and by giving them names you enable her to store away vocabulary that she will later be able to draw upon when she begins to speak.
- Play games with her that involve taking turns. Hand her a rattle and wait for her to hand it back.
- Keep your speech clear and simple. You may automatically pitch your voice higher and speak more slowly to your baby.
- Use gestures to emphasize what you are saying, e.g. hold up her coat as you say, 'Now let's put your coat on'; and do the actions as you say, 'One arm . . . now the other arm.'
- Give your baby plenty of time to process what you are saying.
- Repeat yourself and ask questions, to give your baby the opportunity to remember what you say.
- Don't worry about using 'baby talk'. It helps your baby understand new words and encourages her to try them out.
- Accept her mispronunciations and baby language, and don't overcorrect her or you will discourage her.
- Don't hog the conversation, even if your baby can't talk. Listen and respond to the sounds she makes.
- Emphasize names and objects. Many of her first words will be label words – dog, coat, cup, and so on.
- Keep up a commentary of what you are doing as you go about your daily tasks: 'Now we're going to wash your hands'; 'Here's your bottle', and so on.
- Keep your conversation in the present tense – your baby cannot remember well what happened in the past or anticipate tomorrow.
- Don't worry about using 'good' English – the main thing is to encourage your baby to speak.

When to worry

Most babies start to talk at between nine and 18 months old, so there is no need to be concerned if your baby doesn't say her first word before she is one. Talking depends on hearing, so it is essential that hearing tests are carried out. In most areas your baby will have a routine hearing test at around seven or eight months, and if it appears that she is having hearing difficulties, a repeat test will be performed about a month later. It is vital that any serious hearing loss is picked up before it has the chance to affect a baby's speech and language development.

If your baby appears to be hard of hearing, for instance if she doesn't respond to you when you speak to her softly, especially if you are out of sight, consult your doctor or health visitor. If your baby has a lot of coughs, colds, catarrh or other infections she could experience some difficulty in hearing from time to time. She may also be at risk of hearing problems if:

- You or your husband are hearing-impaired.
- Any other children you have are deaf.
- You have had several miscarriages.
- You had German measles (rubella) during the first three months of pregnancy.
- Your baby was premature or suffered severe lack of oxygen during birth.

None of these mean your baby will necessarily be hard of hearing, but if you suspect that she is having problems, don't hesitate to talk to your doctor or health visitor as there are many ways in which she can be helped.

PLAY

Play isn't an idle occupation for your baby; it is a serious – though hugely enjoyable – business. One of the great joys of parenthood is to join in your child's games. It is fascinating to watch how he practises and develops his skills and abilities through playing.

Play is inextricably linked with your baby's development. By watching your baby and anticipating his needs you will be able to provide him with the right toys and games to extend and foster his growing mastery of his environment. Your baby doesn't need a lot of expensive toys. You will soon learn to spot the play potential in a wide range of household objects. The only rule is that anything you give him to play with should be safe. Watch out for any loose pieces or sharp edges; and don't give him anything so small he could swallow it.

THE FIRST SIX MONTHS: LEARNING ABOUT THE WORLD

During this time your baby is learning about this strange, new place into which he has been born. To do so he uses his senses – seeing, hearing, tasting, smelling, touching. Later, as he gains control of his limbs and hands, he will want games and playthings that provide him with the opportunity to use his body. He also has to learn how to communicate. But above all he has to learn about cause and effect and how the things that he does can affect the world around him.

Your baby will learn best with you as a friend and playmate. Fortunately there is potential for play and learning in all sorts of daily activities. You don't have to deliberately sit and play with your baby all the time, although, of course, you will both enjoy those special times when you are together 'just playing'.

Toys and aids for the first six months		
Baby bouncing chair	Rattles	Soft blocks
Mobiles	Musical toys	Mirror (unbreakable)

Feeding his senses
At first your baby relies entirely on you to provide him with experience of the world.

- Carry him around the house with you and show him interesting things: a picture, an ornament, the way the wind wafts the curtains – the only limit is your imagination. Give him plenty of time to explore what he sees with his eyes, and to take it in. Hold him about 25 cm (10 in.) away from an object, as he focuses best at this distance.
- At first he won't be able to hold his head in mid-line, but will lie with it to one side. Fix brightly coloured postcards or pictures to the side of his cot, crib or pram, so that he can look at them as he lies there. Hang small toys or rattles from the side of his cot. Waft

brightly coloured ribbons or a balloon from side to side as he lies there and watch as he follows it with his eyes.

- Prop him up where he can see you going about your daily tasks. Remember there is no one more interesting and fascinating to your baby than you.

- Your baby loves the movement of the mobile that hangs and swings above his cot, leaves dancing in the wind, bubbles drifting past his eyes. It's up to you to show him how things move. Line up skittles or plastic squash bottles and throw a ball at them. Watch his eyes light up as they topple and fall.

- Suspend interesting objects from a coat hanger above his cot, for example a non-breakable Christmas tree bauble, rattle, cotton reel, yoghurt cartons, pieces of bright, crinkly paper, ribbons, wind chimes. Babies love bright, shiny shapes that catch the light, and bold patterns. Change the objects on the mobile from time to time, as your baby will tire of seeing the same things. Always aim to include some objects that make an interesting noise, as well as things that are good to look at.

- Your baby will be fascinated by the moving reflection in a mirror placed at the side of his cot, or hung from a rod above his crib. But not until the age of six or seven months will he recognize the moving shapes as his own.

- When your baby is about three months old fix a rod or piece of elastic across his cot just within his reach, and thread a wooden spoon, rattle, cotton reel, woollen pom pom and other safe household objects on to it so that he can swipe at them. Change the objects frequently.

- Give him the opportunity to handle and feel different types of material: a silk scarf, a piece of crackly paper, a teaspoon.

- Attach a small toy to a stick and move it slowly across his field of vision.

- Fill a pillow case with crinkly paper, sew it up and place it over the end of your baby's cot. Encourage your baby to kick it and make it rustle. Let him kick against soft blocks too. He is learning that what he does has an effect on the world around him.

- As well as bought rattles there are plenty of everyday objects that can be made to produce fascinating noises. Fill a plastic bottle or other container with dried peas, beans, rice or coins and seal it with tape.

- Firmly sew a couple of bells on to a pair of 'scratch mittens' (the cotton mittens you can buy to prevent your baby scratching his face), put them on him and watch his fascination as his hands start to tinkle! You could make the mittens even more interesting for your baby by embroidering or appliquéing a face on them and making the bell the 'nose'. Babies love to look at faces. Such a toy helps hand-eye co-ordination, and helps him to learn about cause and effect.

- You can add to your baby's enjoyment of smell and taste. Take him for a walk through a rose garden. Sprinkle a few drops of scented oil, such as orange, rose, or lavender, on the radiator in his room. In the summer fill his room with scented flowers such as sweet peas or carnations. Once you start offering him a few solids at around the age of four to six months provide him with a wide variety of tastes.

- Sing to your baby: gentle, soothing lullabies as he is about to go to sleep; boisterous, bouncing rhymes when he is alert and awake.

- At around the age of three months he will start to grasp things deliberately. Provide him with plenty of opportunities to do so. At first he will manage best with lightweight rattles, such as those made of cane or 'lacy' plastic. Later he can progress to a sturdier sort. Look for rattles that provide plenty of interest: different colours, shapes, sounds, holes in which he can poke his fingers. At first he will drop them constantly. Your job is to be patient and keep offering him things to hold and shake. Later on he will explore each object minutely. Everything goes to his mouth, so keep his toys clean, and give them an occasional rinse in sterilizing solution.

Co-ordinating hands and eyes

At around the age of four months your baby begins to co-ordinate his hand and eye movements. For the last month or so he has spent a lot of time gazing at his hands as he held them up in front of his face, clasping and unclasping them. Now he deliberately fixes an object in his gaze and then, constantly checking from eye to hand in order to measure the distance, he reaches out for it. Gradually he becomes more efficient at using his hands. He is able to estimate the distance of an object, then reach out for it surely. As his knowledge becomes more refined he can tell at a glance how far he has to reach. You can help him develop co-ordination by giving him plenty of practice in reaching and grasping, and by making sure he has plenty of different objects to hold. Vary size, shape, weight and texture.

THE SECOND SIX MONTHS: A WORLD OF OBJECTS

During the age of six to 12 months your baby's main interest shifts from people to objects. He is fascinated by things, but he still needs you to provide him with the objects that he will enjoy. Towards the end of this period he starts to be more actively exploratory and will appreciate toys and activities that encourage him to use his body.

Toys and aids for the second six months

Baby bouncer	Plastic and wooden blocks	Paddling pool
Baby walker	Push-and-pull toys	Bucket and spade
Activity centres	Balls of various sizes	Water mill
Bath toys	Suction toys	Posting toys
Stacking toys	Wobbly toys	Books
Jack-in-the-box	Rolling toys	

Exploring together

- During this period your baby learns that things that have gone from sight are nonetheless still there. Now is the time for all those peek-a-boo and hide-and-seek games. Wrap objects in a soft cloth or layers of paper (not stuck down) and let him 'find' them. Cover a small toy with an upturned plastic flowerpot or bucket.

- As he begins to realize that objects have a permanent existence he will enjoy bought toys such as a jack-in-the-box and other pop-up toys.

- Post a set of keys, ping-pong ball, cotton reel or other small object down a long cardboard tube, such as the type used for kitchen foil or film, and watch his delight and surprise when it appears at the other end.

- From the age of six months he will enjoy bathtime. Give him a variety of funnels, plastic containers, spoons, and so on, so that he can learn all the properties of water. Show him how water drips, pours, squelches, splashes, whooshes, trickles. Use the words – he will be fascinated by them and by the way they imitate the sounds made by the water itself. He may even try to say the words himself.

- Your baby will love putting things in a container. There are toys available that enable him to do this, for instance a set of plastic saucepans and various posting toys. Just as effective, however, is a large, plastic ice-cream tub and a selection of household objects. As he fills and empties he is learning how to manipulate a variety of different shapes, sizes and weights.

- As he begins to appreciate the permanence of objects he will enjoy throwing things for you to pick up. He'll never tire of this game – although you probably will – and it will help his manipulative skills. Tie toys to the side of his highchair or pram, so he can retrieve them himself, but don't leave him unsupervised as he could become twisted in the ribbon or string.

- Let him drop things into a container such as a saucepan or biscuit tin that make a noise.

- Your baby loves to copy you. When he is about a year old buy him a few imaginative toys, such as a tea set or a telephone, and encourage him to copy you pouring out the tea or making a phone call. In this way, you will stimulate his imagination and social skills. He may even be ready for a few 'pretend' games; for example, once he is used to using the toy telephone, pick up a banana and pretend it's a telephone receiver. He may think you've gone bananas! On the other hand, he may understand what you are doing and copy you. It's the beginning of thinking about other people's thoughts – a vital social skill.

- By the time he is one he will enjoy simple finger puppets. You can buy a set or make your own, using paper, card or felt. This helps to develop his communication skills as well as improving his manipulative control. You can use finger puppets to chant or sing rhymes such as Two Tall Policemen, Tommy Thumb, and so on (see pages 105–6).

- Balls and rolling toys will help him develop physical skills such as crawling. As well as bought toys, you can use household objects, such as a biscuit tin and washing-up liquid bottle, for him to chase after.

- Encourage your baby's developing memory by ensuring that some things in his life remain constant. If you always sing the same lullaby as you put him to sleep, he will learn to anticipate it. Keep a few familiar soft toys on his windowsill or at the end of his bed, and let him say goodnight to them before you lay him down to sleep. Make games out of his everyday routines: he will come to recognize such phrases as 'Skin a rabbit!' as you pull off his vest, and when he hears it he will raise his arms to help you ease it over his head. Such games are all part of his growing understanding and communication.

- Once your baby can walk he will enjoy push-and-pull toys. There is a variety of toys you can buy, such as a telephone that rolls its eyes and chatters as you pull it along, or a rolling ball on a stick that rattles when you push it. You can improvise many of your own, too: for instance, thread cotton reels on a piece of string or ribbon to make a 'clatterpillar'; fill a large, plastic sweet jar from the confectioners with pasta shells, beans or anything else that makes a noise and fix string to the lid so he can pull it along. Such games will aid his rather unsteady balance and improve his co-ordination and manipulative skills. They also exercise his problem-solving abilities.
- At a year old he will enjoy a few board books with large, clear illustrations. Look at them together and point out the objects. Your baby will also enjoy looking at old catalogues – and it doesn't matter if he tears them. Books help develop his language and his manipulative skills as he works out how to turn the pages one by one.

Songs and action rhymes

Babies are naturally musical. Your baby will gain a range of language and social skills by listening to you sing to him. He will join in by 'singing' and bouncing in time to the rhythm. He is also learning to communicate and take turns. Above all, he is learning the pleasure and fascination of words, and how that pleasure can be shared with others. Repetition of words and actions helps him to anticipate. Forward planning is an important part of understanding and making sense of the world, as it is of language development.

These are just a few tried-and-tested favourites. If you invest in a good nursery rhyme book, you will soon learn many more.

Shoe a Little Horse
Pat the soles of your baby's feet as you say this rhyme.

> Shoe a little horse
> Shoe a little mare
> But let the little colt
> Go bare, bare, bare

Round and Round the Haystack
Most people are familiar with Round and Round the Garden, and if

your baby likes it try this variation. Circle your finger around the palm
of your baby's hand, then walk your finger along the baby's arm and
tickle him under the arm. Your baby learns to anticipate the final
tickle. Learning to assess what is going to happen is an important ability.

> Round and round the haystack
> Runs the little mouse
> One step, two steps
> In her little house

Leg over Leg

Bounce your baby on your foot as you sing this rhyme. When you come
to the word 'jump' give an extra big bounce.

> Leg over leg
> The dog runs to Dover
> When he comes to a stile
> Jump – he goes over

To Market, to Market

Bounce your baby on your knee as you sing this rhyme. He will learn to
listen for the different sounds of the words.

> To market to market
> To buy a fat pig
> Home again, home again
> Jiggety jig

> To market, to market
> To buy a fat hog
> Home again, home again
> Joggety jog

Two Tall Policemen

Use your fingers in order as you repeat the rhyme, or for a variation use
finger puppets.

> Two fine ladies met in a lane (index fingers)
> Bowed most politely (waggle your fingers to the words)
> Bowed once again

How-dya-do, How-dya-do, How-dya-do
Two tall policeman (middle fingers)
Repeat chorus
Two small schoolboys (ring fingers)
Repeat chorus
Two little babies (little fingers)
Repeat chorus

Your baby learns about taking turns and will improve his manipulative skills as he tries to copy you.

Tommy Thumb
Hide each finger behind your back and bring it out as you say the words 'Here I am'. Finally, bring your whole hand out and waggle your fingers.

Tommy Thumb, Tommy Thumb
Where are you?
Here I am, here I am
How do you do
Peter Pointer, Peter Pointer (index finger)
Toby Tall, Toby Tall (middle finger)
Ruby Ring, Ruby Ring (ring finger)
Baby Small, Baby Small (little finger)
Fingers all, Fingers all (all fingers and thumbs)
Where are you?
Here we are, here we are
How do you do

A Mouse Lived in a Little Hole
Shape your left hand into a fist, leaving a narrow hole into which you insert your index finger as you say the words and mime the actions. As you say, 'Out popped he', pull your finger out and waggle it at your baby.

A mouse lived in a little hole
Lived softly in a little hole (said quietly)
When all was quiet
As quiet as can be (whisper the words)
OUT POPPED HE (shout words)

As he becomes familiar with the rhymes, he will remember them and try to join in, so helping him to improve his memory and feel secure.

TYPES OF PLAY

Experts distinguish four main types of play, corresponding to your
baby's main areas of development. These aren't intended to be cut and
dried, some games and activities obviously fit into more than one
category. Below are some suggestions for catering for these four types of
play, although you will think of many more yourself.

Type of play	Purpose it serves	Games, toys, activities
ACTIVE PHYSICAL PLAY	To develop muscles and movement. To develop control, co-ordination and balance. Leads on to sports and active pastimes.	Baby bouncer, bouncing chair, push-and-pull toys, baby walker, push-along truck, rolling toys, balls, climbing over furniture, swing, action songs involving large movements, ride-on toys.
MANIPULATIVE PLAY	To develop finer movements and co-ordination of hands and eyes. Preparation for skill involving fine movements such as feeding, dressing, doing up buttons, drawing, writing.	Rattles, beads, squeaky toys, blocks, balls, board books, catalogues, posting toys, stacking toys, finger games, rhymes.
PRETEND PLAY Most babies do not engage in this sort of play until their second or even third year.	To encourage the development of imagination, vital in planning and understanding the thoughts of others. To help work out emotions. To teach self-awareness.	Simple story books, imitative games, e.g. putting your tongue out and letting him copy you, toy tea set, telephone, messy play, water play, songs and rhymes.

Type of play	Purpose it serves	Games, toys, activities
SOCIAL PLAY	To help emotional development. To teach co-operation, taking turns, sharing and communication with others. To help build up good relationships with others and make friends – all vital skills for when adult.	Any game or activity you share together, playing with other babies, meeting relatives and friends, peek-a-boo, pat-a-cake, and any other games involving taking turns.

Toy safety

- Check all bought toys for safety. Sturdy, well-made toys from a reliable manufacturer are the best as they usually comply with safety regulations. If money is tight, buy a few such toys and improvise the rest from household objects.
- Avoid toys made of thin, hard plastic, as bits can chip off leaving sharp, dangerous edges.
- Inspect toys regularly for breakages, loose parts and sharp or ragged edges.
- Avoid toys with tiny holes that could trap your baby's fingers.
- Make sure that eyes and other small parts are firmly attached to soft toys.
- Don't give your baby objects that contain dye that runs. Ensure that any home-made toys are non-toxic – use a lead-free paint.
- Don't leave him unsupervised.
- Never let your baby play with a plastic bag. Tie plastic carrier bags after use so that your baby cannot put one over his head if he accidentally gets hold of it.
- Watch him carefully if you give him anything made of paper. Everything goes to his mouth, and it could soon get soggy and choke him.
- Avoid giving him toys with long pieces of string attached.
- Always supervise water play. A baby can drown in just 5 cm (2 in.) of water.

Part V

KEEPING SAFE AND WELL

IF YOUR BABY IS ILL

It is an extremely rare baby who doesn't pick up one or two minor ailments during her first year, especially if she has older brothers or sisters.

Breast-feeding will confer some immunity to common ailments during your baby's first few months. After that she begins to build up her own resistance to germs.

If your baby is ill you will usually be able to look after her perfectly safely at home. Use your common sense to anticipate the best way of keeping her comfortable.

Never be afraid to call the doctor if you are worried about your baby, even if you cannot be certain of what is wrong. Most doctors have learnt to trust a mother's instincts and understand their worry and distress over a sick baby.

When to call the doctor

- If your baby loses her appetite and refuses her feeds. Once your baby is on solids loss of appetite is less important than a refusal to drink. A child who has stopped drinking for more than a few hours is in danger of dehydration and should receive urgent medical attention.
- Diarrhoea and vomiting, especially if violent and repeated. Again, the danger is of dehydration – save your baby's nappy and a specimen of vomit to show the doctor.
- If your baby develops a rash that looks like spots of blood under the skin.
- Temperature of over 38°C (100°F).
- Convulsions (fits).
- If your baby has a stiff neck.
- If your baby has laboured breathing.

COMMON ILLNESSES AND MINOR HEALTH WORRIES IN THE FIRST YEAR

Colds A cold is a virus, so it cannot be treated by antibiotics. Although you cannot treat your baby's cold, you can make her comfortable. Raise the head of her cot by placing a couple of books under the legs, to make breathing easier. Never use a pillow for a baby under one year old. If a blocked nose is making feeding miserable ask your doctor for some nose drops to clear her air passages. Don't use these for longer than four days without your doctor's advice as prolonged use could damage her delicate mucous membranes.

Cough Your baby coughs to clear her windpipe of mucus and to stop any infection from spreading further down her bronchial tubes. It is therefore inadvisable to suppress a cough with a linctus. Prop up the head of her cot, as above, and make sure she has plenty to drink. If the cough is unusually severe or long-lasting consult your doctor.

Cradle cap This is the yellowish-brown crusty scale that forms on your baby's scalp. Although it looks unpleasant it is not harmful and is not caused by poor hygiene. Try rubbing in a little baby oil or olive oil into your baby's scalp and leaving overnight to soften the scales. Next morning comb her hair and wash with a gentle baby shampoo. If this doesn't work there are special shampoos and gels available to treat the cradle cap. If the cradle cap becomes severe or the skin underneath it seems sore, see the doctor.

Croup The characteristic 'crowing' noise made by a baby who has croup is not a disease in itself, but a symptom. It may be caused by a foreign body being stuck in her windpipe or, more usually, by a swelling and narrowing of the windpipe as it passes through the voice box, as a

---

Taking your baby's temperature

If your baby has a temperature she will feel hot and dry, and may seem drowsy or irritable. The easiest way to take her temperature is to use a heat strip, available from a chemist, which you press against her forehead; if she has a temperature it changes colour. The method is not quite as accurate as using a conventional thermometer, but it is less trouble with a wriggling baby. If you have been told to use a traditional glass thermometer, don't ever put it in your baby's mouth as she could crunch it. A digital thermometer is very convenient for taking a baby's temperature. Simply hold it under her arm for a few minutes and wait for it to bleep before taking the reading.

After your baby is six months old you can bring down her temperature by sponging her with tepid water. Keep her in an even temperature and don't bundle her up in lots of clothes and blankets. A nappy and vest are probably sufficient.

result of infection. It sounds most alarming, but try not to panic as it will only make your baby more agitated. Moist, warm air is the best cure, so boil a kettle and let its steam evaporate into the bedroom, or take your baby into the bathroom and switch on a hot shower. Hold her upright and speak to her calmly. Croup can be dangerous to a very small baby, so you should call the doctor.

Diarrhoea Loose stools are usually unimportant, but if the diarrhoea comes on suddenly and violently, and especially if it is green, recurrent and accompanied by vomiting or a high temperature, your baby could have a gastrointestinal infection. This can be extremely serious in a young baby, as she can quickly become dehydrated. Consult the doctor immediately. Your doctor will usually prescribe a special rehydrating fluid, consisting of glucose and essential mineral salts, to restore your baby's body chemical balance. Use disposable nappies and seal each one in a polythene bag as soon as you remove it. Keep your baby off cow's milk and solid food until the diarrhoea has cleared up, and make sure she has plenty to drink.

Hygiene rules if a member of the family has diarrhoea

Diarrhoea can spread like wildfire among the members of a family. The best protection of all is to breast-feed your baby, as breast milk lines your baby's gut against the germs that cause gastric infection and helps her to withstand it. Since diarrhoea is potentially so serious for a young baby, you should be scrupulously clean if you or any other members of the family have a tummy upset.

- Always wash your hands after using the lavatory.
- Wash your hands before meals.
- Wash your hands before preparing your baby's feed.
- Never leave meat uncovered in the kitchen.
- Avoid leaving frozen chicken uncovered in the kitchen, where it could contaminate other food.
- Cover any cuts, spots or boils, and if a member of the family is suffering from any skin infection, don't let him or her handle the baby's food.

Earache It is difficult to know if your baby has earache since she can't tell you. However, you may suspect it if she holds her ear, rubs it or seems to be off-colour or in pain, especially if she is running a temperature of 38°C (100°F) or more. To relieve the pain place a warmed towel or nappy against her ear and give her a dose of paracetamol syrup. Earache may be caused by a middle ear infection following a cold or measles, and the doctor may prescribe antibiotics. Once your baby has recovered she should have her hearing checked to ensure that it has returned to normal. Any discharge from the ear is abnormal and you should take your baby to see the doctor immediately.

Eczema Infantile eczema is fairly common. It usually starts some time after your baby is three months old. The first sign may be a red, scaly, weeping patch on her face. The eczema may spread to other areas, particularly in the creases of elbows and knees. Although it looks unsightly it is not harmful, and unless your baby seems distressed by it (it can be extremely itchy) there is no need for treatment. Dress your baby in cotton clothing, keep her fingernails short and ask the chemist to recommend a soothing cream.

If your baby seems very uncomfortable and the eczema weeps the doctor may be willing to prescribe a steroid ointment or cream to use sparingly. Most babies with infantile eczema grow out of it by the age of three or four. Breast-fed babies are less likely to suffer from eczema, as it is commonly caused by a cow's milk allergy. If the eczema is severe the doctor may suggest you change to a non-dairy-based baby milk. Biological washing powder is sometimes a cause – use a gentle soap powder and make sure you thoroughly rinse all your baby's laundry. Soap and water may aggravate the eczema, so cleanse your baby's skin with a mild baby lotion instead.

Fever A fever is not an illness as such but a sign of infection caused by a virus or bacteria. Normal body temperature is 35.5–37°C (96–98.4°F). If your baby's temperature rises to 38°C (100°F) or over, call the doctor.

Fits (convulsions) A baby suffering a fit goes pale, her body twitches then becomes stiff, her limbs may shake, and she may foam at the mouth, before she goes floppy and falls asleep. Such fits are most commonly caused by a high temperature (febrile convulsions). Some babies seem prone to them but usually grow out of them by the age of four or five. If your baby has a fit lay her on her side and sponge her with lukewarm water to cool her down. Call the doctor. If your baby has a tendency to febrile convulsions you should try to prevent her becoming

too hot if she has an infection, such as a cold, cough or earache. Keep
her in just a light cotton vest and make sure the room is cool. Tepid
sponging, as described, will help keep her cool, and a dose of
paracetamol syrup will reduce her temperature. More rarely, fits can be
a result of epilepsy, which can be effectively treated.

Hernia This is a bulge caused by underlying tissues breaking through a
weakness in the muscle wall. Many babies have an umbilical hernia,
which usually disappears of its own accord as the muscles grow stronger
within the first year or two of life.

Another sort of hernia is an inguinal hernia, which shows itself as a
lump in your baby's groin. It most commonly affects baby boys. Such a
hernia can become strangulated, so you should consult your doctor if
you suspect your baby is suffering from one. Your baby will usually need
a simple, small operation to correct it.

Jaundice Many babies develop this yellow skin colouring during the
first few days of life. It arises because a baby's immature liver is unable
to process bilirubin, a yellow pigment produced by the breakdown of
the red blood cells. A baby who is jaundiced may be sleepy and slow to
feed. Usually jaundice is not serious and clears up without treatment.
Sometimes it may be treated by placing your baby under a special light
(phototherapy), to help disperse the pigment, and in very extreme
cases a blood transfusion may be necessary. Jaundice is more common
in premature babies.

Possetting Some babies regularly bring up a little of their feed, which
is not harmful and your baby will grow out of it. Handle her gently after
feeds, and avoid bringing her to an upright position abruptly. Protect
your and her clothing with a muslin nappy. And lie her on her side so
that if she does regurgitate a little of her feed it will simply dribble
away. You may like to protect the top of her cot by lying her on a
muslin nappy, or slip a pillow case over the mattress, which you can
turn round and turn over if she messes it.

If your baby vomits forcefully, or if she has diarrhoea and a
temperature, consult the doctor without delay.

Prickly heat Your baby develops itchy red spots when she becomes
overheated. It is not harmful, but you can help make her more

comfortable by giving her a cool bath and applying some calamine lotion or cream on the affected areas. Take care not to overdress your baby in warm weather, and choose cotton rather than synthetic fabrics to prevent her becoming too hot.

Rashes New babies are especially prone to rashes, most of which are not important and clear up without treatment after a day or so. Relieve discomfort by applying a soothing lotion or cream such as calamine. Any rash which goes septic or becomes blistered should be seen by a doctor. Don't use anti-histamine sprays or creams without a doctor's advice as you could set up an allergic reaction. A rash could indicate an infectious illness (see page 117). In this case your baby will probably seem unwell and may be running a fever. Consult your doctor.

Your baby will be exceptionally lucky if she manages to escape the odd bout of nappy rash, especially if the weather is hot. Use a one-way nappy liner and clean her carefully at each change. If the nappy rash weeps it could indicate a type of dermatitis or an infection. See your doctor.

Snuffles Some babies snuffle a lot, because of their narrow nasal passages. Usually as the passages expand towards the end of the first year the snuffliness wears off.

Sore creases The area behind your baby's ears, under her arms and chin, and the creases of her groin may be prone to soreness especially in summer. Give her plenty of warm baths, and apply a protective cream or a light sprinkling of talc. Avoid tight clothes and synthetic fabrics.

Squint Most babies appear to squint until the age of three months, because their eyes are not yet co-ordinated. However, a squint after this age should be reported to the doctor as it could indicate that the eye muscles are not working as they should and need to be corrected. A squint is usually treated by putting a pad over the baby's good eye in order to encourage the muscles of the other eye to work correctly.

Sticky eye Wipe your baby's eyes with cool boiled water, using a separate swab for each eye and working from the bridge of her nose outwards. If this treatment doesn't clear it up, your baby could have an eye infection for which your doctor can prescribe drops or an ointment.

If one eye is often sticky, especially if it seems to water a lot, your baby could have a blocked tear duct, which usually sorts itself out during the first year without the need for treatment. If the problem persists your baby may need a small operation to clear the blockage.

Thrush If your baby's tongue, gums and the inside of her mouth are covered in thick, creamy white patches that cannot be rubbed off, and if she seems to find feeding painful, she may have thrush. It is caused by a yeast infection and may be a result of incompetent sterilization of equipment, or she could have picked it up from your vagina during birth. The doctor can prescribe special drops that will clear it up quickly.

Vomiting Proper vomiting – as opposed to a small amount of regurgitation after a feed – is a serious symptom in a young baby. It can be a sign of other infections such as tonsillitis, ear or urinary infection, or a gastric infection. If your baby vomits and seems unwell, especially if she also has diarrhoea and a temperature, consult your doctor without delay.

If your baby has not opened her bowels for 24 hours and is vomiting, she could have an obstruction of the gut. Again, consult your doctor.

Another type of vomiting is caused by pyloric stenosis, when the tube leading out of your baby's stomach becomes swollen and obstructed. The condition starts about two to three weeks after birth and affects more boys than girls. The baby vomits violently and forcefully after each feed. If the doctor diagnoses pyloric stenosis your baby will need a small operation to correct it.

Wax in the ears Some babies are more prone to producing a lot of wax than others. There is no need to do anything about it. Simply clean the outside of your baby's ear with a twist of cotton wool or tissue. Never poke anything inside your baby's ears or use ear drops unless they are prescribed.

COMMON CHILDHOOD INFECTIOUS ILLNESSES

Your baby's natural immunity, passed on from you through the placenta, will usually protect her from the common childhood illnesses during the first six months of life. Breast-feeding also offers some protection, and if you breast-feed for longer than six months she may be protected accordingly.

The common childhood illnesses tend to run in epidemics. If your baby mixes with many other children, and if you have older children who may bring back germs from school or play group, she may be more susceptible. Most of these illnesses have an incubation period between the time of exposure to the infection and the development of the illness. During this time your baby may seem off-colour and fractious. If you suspect your baby has one of these illnesses call your doctor.

Many of these illnesses can now be prevented by immunization (see page 124). It is important to take advantage of the immunization programme, so that your baby is protected as much as possible.

COMMON CHILDHOOD ILLNESSES

Illness	Incubation Time	Signs & Symptoms
Chickenpox	14–21 days	Sore throat, temperature, followed by rash of spots on chest, abdomen, thighs, face, scalp, legs and arms. At first the spots are raised and red; they then blister and form scabs, which drop off. The spots are very itchy.
German measles (rubella)	14–21 days	Sore throat and runny nose, swollen glands behind ears and nape of neck. Pink rash or fine, unraised spots that join together to give a flushed appearance, starting on the forehead and spreading over rest of body.

IF YOUR BABY IS ILL

Giving medicine

- Follow the doctor's instructions precisely – never give more or less than the stated dose and complete the full course of any antibiotics prescribed.
- Measure the correct amount in a spoon or use one of the special calibrated medicine spoons available from a chemist. Sit your baby on your lap, pull her chin down so that her mouth is open and pour the medicine as far back into her mouth as you can.
- After giving the medicine you can give her a drink or a breast-feed to 'take the taste away' and comfort her.
- Your baby may take medicine more easily from a dropper or from your finger. Dip a clean finger in the medicine and let her suck it off.

Treatment	*Duration of Infection*
Keep your baby cool and comfortable. Give her frequent warm baths with bicarbonate of soda added to soothe itching and apply calamine lotion or cream to the spots. Keep your baby's fingernails short – if she scratches off the scabs she may develop permanent scars. Your doctor may prescribe a mild sedative to relieve itching if your baby is unduly troubled by it.	From one or two days before spots appear until they have all formed scabs.
No treatment, but **keep your baby away from anyone who is pregnant.**	For as long as rash remains.

COMMON CHILDHOOD ILLNESSES

Illness	Incubation Time	Signs & Symptoms
Measles	10–15 days	Bad cold and cough, raised temperature. Puffy, red, watery eyes. The inside of the mouth is inflamed and there may be white spots inside the cheeks. After three or four days red, blotchy rash starts behind ears and hairline and spreads to body.
Mumps	14–28 days	Slightly raised temperature. Swollen glands in front of and below ear. Face may appear misshapen and baby may have difficulty swallowing.
Roseola infantum	7–21 days	High temperature, followed by small, flat, pink spots, similar to German measles rash.
Scarlet fever	2–5 days	Fever, sore throat, vomiting. Tonsils become swollen and inflamed, tongue furry and white with red dots. A day or so later fine, red rash on neck, spreading to rest of body. May scale after it disappears.
Whooping cough	7–14 days	Slight cold, runny nose, mild temperature, developing into severe cough, which may involve 'whoop'. Baby often vomits after fit of coughing. Some babies don't 'whoop' and may turn blue or even have a fit.

Treatment	Duration of Infection
Paracetamol syrup, tepid sponging to reduce fever and keep your baby comfortable. Plenty of drinks. Your doctor may prescribe antibiotics to try to forestall secondary infections such as ear or eye infections, which can be a complication of measles.	Five days before rash appears to five days after fever appears.
Plenty of drinks, and cold, soft foods if your baby is on solids. Avoid anything acid.	Two days before swellings, until they disappear.
Treat fever with paracetamol syrup and tepid sponging.	Not known.
Antibiotics, rest.	From onset until throat is clear.
Antibiotics may be given in early stages or late depending on lung complications. Sedatives to help baby sleep. Raise head of cot to ease breathing, and hold baby upright when she coughs.	About a month from two days before cough sets in.

Survival tips for when your baby is ill

- Cut down on housework.
- Accept offers of help.
- Make use of convenience foods until she gets a bit better.
- If she is wakeful at night, move into her room for the duration of the illness.
- Catch up on rest during the day when she sleeps.

TEETHING

Your baby's 20 milk teeth are already in his gums when he is born. In fact, some babies even have a tooth at birth! This tooth is additional to his other milk teeth and will usually be removed. Gradually, over the next couple of years, the teeth will push their way through his gums. The exact timing varies – some babies cut their first tooth at around three months, others not until the end of their first year – and depends on your baby's individual biological clock.

The average age for the first tooth to appear is six months when one of the two middle, biting teeth (incisors) in the bottom gum pushes its way to the surface. About a month later one of the top, middle, biting teeth comes through, and two or three months after that the teeth on either side of these appear. By the time your baby is a year old he will probably have six teeth.

Does teething hurt?

No one is quite sure how painful teething is for babies. Some babies seem to sail through teething with little or no discomfort. Others become irritable, rub their gums and dribble. The dribbling often causes a red teething rash, and your baby may have difficulty settling at night because of the discomfort.

Some experts think that teething lowers the baby's resistance, so laying him open to other infections – which is why so many babies seem to go through a patch of minor illness when they are teething. Others believe that it is just coincidence – given that your baby will be coming in contact with various ailments at the time his natural immunity is wearing down – and that any illness he contracts just happens to occur at the same time as he is teething.

ERUPTION OF
MILK TEETH IN THE
ORDER IN WHICH
THEY APPEAR

UPPER

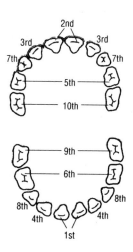

LOWER

Whichever side you come down on, one thing is for certain: teething does not cause diarrhoea, sickness, high temperature, fits or loss of appetite. These are all serious symptoms and if your baby develops any of them you should contact your doctor.

How you can help your baby

If teething is causing your baby discomfort, give him plenty of hard things to chew on: a teething ring or shapes, a peeled carrot, slice of apple, hard rusk, and so on. Always make sure you stay with your baby while he is chewing on these foods in case he chokes. Provide him with plenty of cooling drinks, from a cup if he finds sucking from bottle or breast uncomfortable. Wrap an ice cube in a clean nappy liner or piece of muslin, and apply it to his gums, or rub them with a teething gel available from the chemist. If your baby is having trouble sleeping, a dose of paracetamol syrup will help relieve pain and allow him to drift off. If teething problems persist for longer than a couple of days when he cuts his tooth, consult your doctor.

Looking after your baby's teeth

It is never too early to start caring for your baby's teeth. Avoid sweet drinks and sticky foods. Give him water to drink after his meals to help wash any food residue from his teeth and gums. Ask your doctor or dentist whether he recommends fluoride drops or tablets, to help strengthen the teeth and make them resistant to decay. The best way to beat tooth decay is to avoid letting your baby develop a sweet tooth. He will come to appreciate the natural sweetness of fruits and vegetables if you don't give him sugary biscuits or sweets.

Even though your child will lose his milk teeth when his permanent ones come through, it is important to keep his first teeth healthy, to keep the spaces free for his second teeth and to ensure proper development of his jaw. You can clean his teeth by wiping them with a piece of muslin after he has eaten. Later on, when he is about a year old, provide him with a soft toothbrush and let him copy you cleaning your teeth. It won't be effective at first, of course, so you will need to continue to clean them for him until he is at least four or five.

IMMUNIZATION

Immunization involves giving your child a special vaccine in order to stimulate her body's defence system to produce antibodies. When your child encounters the illness against which she has been immunized, her immune system protects her from it, or at least ensures that if she does catch it it will be in a mild form.

Immunization is important not only to protect your baby, but to keep disease levels low in the community at large and prevent the spread of infection. When immunization rates fall there are flare-ups of epidemics; since some parents have failed to have their children immunized against whooping cough there has been a resurgence of this childhood illness.

Your baby is eligible for free immunization against diphtheria, tetanus, polio, whooping cough, measles, mumps and rubella (German measles). It is important to take advantage of immunization against all these illnesses, although in special circumstances you may be advised against the whooping cough or measles vaccine.

Your doctor or health visitor will tell you when your baby is due to be

IMMUNIZATION SCHEDULE

The precise timing of the various vaccinations may vary slightly from
one area to another. A typical schedule is as follows.

Age	Disease	Side effects if any	When not advisable
3 months	Diphtheria, tetanus, whooping cough (triple vaccine)	Slight redness and swelling at injection site	If baby is unwell with a temperature. Whooping cough vaccine is inadvisable where there is: • A history of fits • Brain damage or nervous system disorder • Epilepsy in a close family member
3 months	Polio (oral vaccine)	None	No instances
5 months	Booster dose of triple vaccine and polio	None	Any severe reaction to a previous dose
9–12 months	Booster dose of triple vaccine and polio	None	Any severe reaction to a previous dose
Some time in second year	Measles, mumps and rubella (German measles) – MMR	Redness and swelling. Occasionally rash 10–14 days after injection	Virtually no instances. If baby suffers convulsions, the doctor will probably give a special protective injection at the same time to prevent complications

immunized. Make sure you keep all appointments unless your child is unwell, in which case your doctor may postpone giving the vaccination.

　　Any side effects from the immunization are usually mild. If your baby does have a reaction, it usually takes the form of a slight swelling at the site of the injection, and she may appear a little off-colour.

Triple vaccine

This is a course of three injections given at intervals during the first year against diphtheria, tetanus and whooping cough (pertussis). Whooping cough can be extremely serious in a small baby. A minute proportion of babies suffer a very severe reaction to the whooping cough vaccine; those with disorders of the nervous system or who suffer from epilepsy or fits should not receive it. Always ask your doctor for advice on the whooping cough vaccine and do not simply make your own decision. Your doctor will advise against the vaccine if it would be unwise for your baby.

Polio vaccine

This is given by mouth. Delay the vaccination if your baby has diarrhoea or vomiting.

ENSURING YOUR BABY'S SAFETY

Your baby cannot protect himself and, as he gets older and more active, he can easily encounter danger if you are not on your guard. The secret is to stay one step ahead of your baby's developing abilities and to anticipate the possible danger spots in your home.

BIRTH TO SIX MONTHS

At first your baby has no control over his body. His basic reflexes help to protect him from harm, but you need to protect him from risks that arise from his age and inexperience.

Temperature

Your baby cannot control his body temperature easily, so you must ensure that he does not become either overheated or too cold. If your baby was born early or was low birth weight he is particularly prone to the effects of cold. Make sure the temperature in his room does not fall below 21°C (70°F). Once he has reached 3.6 kg (8 lb.) in weight you can safely let the temperature drop a little, so long as it does not fall below 16°C (60°F) at night. Make sure his cot is not placed in a draught.

Avoiding sunburn

Your baby's skin is thinner and more delicate than that of an adult, so even if he has a dark skin tone you must ensure that he is not exposed to direct sunlight.

- Use a parasol or canopy on his pram or pushchair.
- Guard his skin with a cream that provides a high protection factor sunscreen.
- Protect his head with a sun hat.
- Dress him in a long-sleeved T-shirt or shirt to protect his arms.
- Don't let an older baby or toddler play in the midday sun.
- Give him plenty of fluids to drink when the weather is hot.
- Let him play in a paddling pool to help keep him cool, but never leave him there unattended.

If your baby gets sunburnt

Sunburn only becomes apparent a few hours after exposure. If he is suffering from sunburn:

- Consult the doctor.
- Bathe your baby in lukewarm water.
- Apply calamine lotion or cream to ease the pain.
- Offer plenty to drink.
- Give a dose of paracetamol syrup to help relieve pain.
- Keep the burn covered until it has healed.

Breathing

Your baby has a basic instinct that enables him to keep his airways clear, but he cannot breathe through his mouth. Never give him a pillow as he could bury his head in it and suffocate. If you use pillows to prop him up in his pram, choose the ventilated kind. If you provide him with a carrying nest to keep him snug and warm, choose one without a hood, elastic or cords, and put a rolled towel or blanket in the bottom of the nest so that he cannot slip down it and bury his head.

In his pram
- Check the pram regularly for loose, worn or damaged parts.
- Check brakes regularly. Never park the pram on a steep hill.
- As soon as your baby can sit up make sure he wears a safety harness.
- Protect him from cats and insects by using a cat net.
- Don't leave him unattended in his pram outside shops.
- If you use a toddler seat don't leave him on it unattended, as he could bounce and upturn the pram.

In his crib or cot
- Don't put him down to sleep with his bib on.
- Don't use loose sheets. Choose fitted bottom sheets or cover the mattress with a pillow case.
- Lay him on his side to avoid the danger of choking if he vomits while lying on his back.
- If you use an electric blanket or hot-water bottle remove it before putting your baby down.
- Check that the spaces between the bars are small enough to prevent him from trapping his head in them or slipping out between them – not less than 2.5 cm (1 in.) and not more than 6 cm (2½ in.).
- Check that there are no gaps between cot side and mattress.
- If you have bought second-hand and are re-painting, make sure the paint you use is lead-free. Remove any decorative transfers, and check for loose, worn or damaged parts and replace them.

SIX MONTHS TO A YEAR

From now on your baby is an active explorer. By six months he can roll over, so never leave him lying on a high surface such as a bed, table or changing unit. His new-found ability to grasp and handle objects increases the risks of accidents too, so be on your guard and when you sit with him, push all cups of tea and hot things well out of his reach. Check your house for hazards (see guide over next few pages), and check all toys for small, loose or breakable parts. Never leave your baby alone where he could fall. Baby walkers can be a source of accidents: never leave him unattended in one, and don't use it upstairs or near an open fire. Protect fires with a fireguard.

Towards the end of your baby's first year he develops a fine pincer grip. Check the floor for small objects such as hair grips, coins, paper clips, small toys or parts from an older child's toys. Now is the time to go through your house room by room and check for safety.

Kitchen

- Keep all cleaning fluids locked away, preferably high up and never in the cupboard under the sink.
- Make sure your cooker is stable.
- Protect the cooker with a guard, and when cooking make sure you turn all saucepan handles inwards.
- When working in the kitchen it may be advisable to put your baby in a playpen to keep him out of harm's way.
- Never leave your baby alone in the kitchen even for a second.
- Always wipe up any grease or spills immediately.
- Check floor tiles or vinyl for loose edges or corners and stick them down.
- Never leave pet food on the floor in the kitchen – it acts like a magnet to a crawling baby and can be a source of harmful bacteria.
- Place electrical appliances well back on the work surface.

Kitchen hygiene

The kitchen can be a germ trap if you are not careful.

- Wash the floor every day using disinfectant and paying special attention to corners and the areas beneath work surfaces and appliances where food and debris easily collect.
- Unfinished bottles or feeder cups of milk should be disposed of immediately.
- Cool leftovers quickly, cover and store in fridge. Keep leftover cooked meats and poultry, eggs and egg produce, shellfish and rice well covered and away from raw meat.
- Keep a special chopping board and knife for raw meat.
- Thoroughly defrost and cook any meat that has been frozen. You need to be especially careful with frozen chicken, as it can be a breeding ground for the salmonella bacteria.
- Remove any animal bowls from the floor as soon as your pet has finished eating.
- Keep all pet litter trays outside the house.
- Keep waste bins out of the way of the baby. Use the type of bin with a twist-on lid rather than a swing or pedal bin.
- Avoid tea towels as they are teeming with germs. Wash crockery in very hot water and leave to air dry. If you must use tea towels, replace them daily.

- Make sure electric flexes are short or coiled. Avoid leaving flexes trailing.
- The minute you finish using the iron switch it off and put it somewhere safe to cool down.
- Keep sharp knives out of your baby's reach.
- Avoid tablecloths.
- Lock freezer, tumble dryer, washing machine and any other large appliances that your baby could crawl into.
- Put safety locks on any doors leading to the outside.
- If you have a microwave have it serviced regularly.
- Keep plastic bags out of your baby's reach – or, better still, dispose of them. If you store them for reuse tie them in a knot or cut holes in the bottom of them.
- Never fill a chip pan more than a third full of oil. If it catches fire cover with a lid, damp towel or safety blanket. Never douse a flaming chip pan with water or try to carry it out of the house.
- Keep a safety blanket or fire extinguisher in the kitchen.
- Never pass hot food or drinks over your baby's head.

Living room
- Remove heavy and breakable objects from low tables.
- Remove any poisonous houseplants.
- Make sure all fires are guarded with a nursery fireguard, which is secured to the wall.
- Check electrical appliances regularly for faults and avoid having flexes that run around the edges of a room.
- Protect electrical sockets with socket covers when not in use.
- Never overload electrical sockets.
- Don't balance ashtrays on arms of chairs. Avoid smoking when your baby is in the room.
- Clear away ash and cigarette stubs immediately, in case your baby finds them and puts them in his mouth.
- Make sure any bookcases and free-standing furniture are stable.
- Never dry clothes or nappies over a heater.
- Avoid paraffin heaters. If you have one, make sure that it is secured to the floor and serviced regularly.
- Keep matches and lighters well out of your baby's reach.
- Repair loose or worn rugs or carpets.
- Make sure there are non-slip mats under any loose rugs.

- Replace any glass doors or low-level windows with safety glass that does not shatter.
- Cover non-safety glass with safety film available from DIY shops or glass merchants, and stick transfers on it to make sure glass is visible.
- Keep sewing and knitting materials out of the way.
- Don't leave hot or alcoholic drinks where your child can reach them.
- Keep television, video recorder and hi-fi out of reach if you can.

Hall and stairs
- Make sure any doors leading outside are locked.
- Fit safety locks to windows.
- Always make sure the door is closed after you have answered it, or after you have been out to fetch something – your baby could crawl out into the road.
- Don't put glass doors at the bottom of stairs.
- Make sure stair carpets are firmly fixed and repair them immediately if they become loose.
- Make sure banisters are secure and have narrow gaps between rails. Board up horizontal banisters so your baby cannot climb up them. Board up spaces on open-tread staircases.
- Keep stairs well lit and free from toys that could trip you up when you come down carrying your baby.
- Protect stairs at top and bottom with a safety gate. The type that opens and closes is the most practical.

Bathroom and lavatory
- Don't leave your baby alone in the bath for a second, as he can drown in a surprisingly small amount of water.
- Run cold water into the bath before hot, and always test the temperature of the water on your wrist before putting your baby in it.
- Place a non-slip mat on the bottom of the bath, unless it has a built-in non-slip surface.
- Wrap a nappy or towel around the hot tap to prevent your baby from burns.
- Cover heated towel rails with a towel.
- Keep perfumes, cosmetics and medical equipment in a locked cabinet.

- Never transfer medicines from a childproof container into another bottle or jar.
- Don't mix bleach and other toilet cleaners; the resulting fumes may be lethal. Store toilet and bathroom cleaners well out of your baby's reach.
- Dispose of old medicines by flushing them down the lavatory.
- Use talc sparingly – if your baby inhales the powder it could block his air passages.
- Use a large, firm sponge when bathing your baby. Natural sponges can disintegrate and cause your baby to choke if he sucks on them.
- Fix a thermostat to your shower unit, to avoid burning.

Bedroom

- Don't leave your baby lying alone on a changing unit or bed.
- If your baby sleeps in your bed make sure it is safe and never leave him alone in it.
- Fix safety locks to windows.
- Never leave an electric or other fire within reach of your baby's cot.
- Protect hot radiators with a blanket or towel.
- Never place your baby's cot directly beneath a window.
- Remove bedside lamps, which could be pulled over.
- Store toys low down, so your baby is not tempted to climb to reach them.

Garden

- Check garden for poisonous plants or shrubs, such as laburnum, deadly nightshade, yew, privet, lily of the valley, hydrangea, and remove them if possible.
- Make sure all gates are locked high up.
- Check boundaries for gaps in fences or hedging.
- Cover all sandpits.
- Bury any pet droppings.
- Keep weedkillers and other garden chemicals locked away.
- Don't use lawnmowers, hedge clippers and other garden power tools when your baby is around.
- Check garden play equipment for wear and tear.
- Never store garden chemicals in containers such as lemonade bottles.
- Don't leave paddling pool with water in it. Always supervise any water play.

- Never light a bonfire with paraffin or petrol. Avoid having fires when your baby is around.
- Sheath any sharp blades, such as shears, secateurs, and so on, and store them out of your baby's reach.

In the car
- Your baby should always travel in a special car safety seat, or harnessed in his carrycot, which should be attached to the back seat by special fixings. Check out local loan schemes for child car seats. In some areas hospitals and local groups hire out car seats at a reasonable rate.
- Fit car safety locks to all doors.
- Don't leave your baby alone in a locked car.
- Don't drive when you are tired or under stress.
- If you are ever in a car accident make sure the car seat and safety fixings are checked by a garage – they may need refitting.

Home first aid kit
Keep a first aid kit, sealed and out of the way for use in an emergency. Replace items as they are used. Useful items include:

- Sterile gauze pads
- Plasters and adhesive tape in a variety of sizes and shapes
- Elastic bandages and gauze bandage in several widths
- Scissors
- Cotton wool
- Cotton buds
- Thermometer or heat strip
- 5 ml medicine spoon
- Tweezers
- Sharp needle and box of matches
- Calamine lotion
- Safety pins
- Pain killers and paracetamol syrup
- Eyebath

Keep a good basic first aid book with the kit, together with the telephone numbers of your doctor, chemist and a 24-hour taxi service. If you leave your baby with a babysitter make sure he or she knows where to find the first aid kit.

IF AN ACCIDENT HAPPENS

You won't be able to prevent your child having the occasional minor injury or accident, however assiduously you watch him. Most minor injuries don't need special treatment, and your main job as a parent is to comfort and reassure. There is a good deal to be said for 'kissing something better'.

In the case of more serious accidents the secret is to be prepared. The following hints will act as a reminder, but all parents could benefit from a proper first aid course like those run by organizations such as St John Ambulance and the Red Cross.

Falls

If your baby has a bad fall the danger is of concussion. There may be signs immediately after the fall or at any time over the subsequent couple of days. Watch out for:

- Drowsiness
- Vomiting
- Fits
- Blood or clear fluid from nose, ear or mouth
- Pallor
- Headache
- Confusion

If any of these signs appears, lay your baby down on his side and call the doctor or an ambulance. If your baby loses consciousness even for a few seconds when he falls, call for medical assistance.

Choking

If your baby chokes he will probably cough or cry hard, which is more effective in clearing the obstruction than anything you can do. However, if he cannot breathe or cough lay him face down over your arm so that his head is lower than his chest. Support his head with your hand and strike him quickly four times between the shoulder blades, using the heel of your hand.

Turn him over, supporting his body between your forearms as you do so, so that he is lying on his back with his head hanging lower than his body. Put two fingertips on his chest between but just below his nipples and press firmly and quickly four times. Repeat this process until he stops choking.

If he stops breathing lay him on the floor. Place one hand on his forehead and the other below his neck and tilt the head back. Take a deep breath and blow very gently into his mouth and nose. Watch to see if his chest rises. When it does take your mouth away and finish breathing out. Watch to see his chest fall, then take another breath in and repeat. Never blow hard or you could damage his tiny lungs. The rate should be about 24 breaths a minute. Once he has started breathing take him to the hospital casualty department as quickly as you can.

Burns and scalds

Prompt first aid to tissue damage should be carried out straight away. For minor burns or scalds (measuring under 5 cm/2 in. across and covering less than 10 per cent of the body), cool the burnt area quickly by holding it under cold running water or immersing it in a basin or sink of cold water. Continue for five minutes, then gently pat dry and cover with a loose dressing. Seek medical attention for deep burns, for burns that blister, or if your baby is suffering from shock.

- Don't remove clothing that is stuck to burnt area.
- Don't put butter or grease on the burn.
- Don't put pressure on a burn.
- Don't burst blisters or remove peeling skin.
- If in doubt take your baby to hospital.

Cuts and grazes

If the cut or graze is small you can safely treat it at home. Wash your hands thoroughly, then wash the wound with soap and water to clean it. Remove any particles, splinters or scraps of dirt with tweezers if necessary but don't remove large objects or glass that is deeply embedded. Flush the wound with warm running water and pat gently dry with a piece of lint or cotton cloth such as a handkerchief. If the edges of the cut are gaping press them together and apply an appropriate dressing. When it is time for the plaster to be removed soak it first in a little baby oil. Inspect the wound from time to time for signs of infection, and if you see redness, swelling or red streaks leading from the wound consult your doctor.

If the injury is more than superficial, if bleeding doesn't stop quickly, or the baby seems to be suffering from shock, take him to hospital.

Electric shock

If the baby is still in contact with the electric current, switch it off by turning off the main circuit breaker or fuse for the whole house, which is situated in your mains fuse box. If this is not possible stand on a thick newspaper or rubber mat and use a wooden pole such as a broom handle to push him away from the current. Don't use bare hands or you will become part of the circuit yourself. Call for medical attention immediately. If the baby is not breathing, carry out mouth-to-mouth resuscitation as for choking (see page 135).

Poisoning

Phone the casualty unit at your local hospital immediately, or if you don't have their number dial 999. Dilute the poison by giving him a couple of glasses of milk or water to drink. Don't make him vomit without advice, as corrosive substances can cause burns of the gullet and digestive passages as they are regurgitated. Take the poison container, plant or any other clue to identification of the poison with you to the hospital, and save any vomit to be tested by collecting it in a bowl or plastic bag.

Do NOT make your baby vomit if he has swallowed:

Strong acid or alkali substances such as:

- ammonia,
- bleach,
- dishwasher detergent,
- drain or lavatory cleaners,
- oven cleaner,
- metal cleaner,
- rust remover

Petroleum-like products such as:

- floor or furniture polish or wax,
- petrol,
- paraffin,
- lighter fluid,
- paint thinner,
- turps

Drowning

Pull the baby out of the water, holding him with his head down to allow the water to drain out. Carry out mouth-to-mouth resuscitation as for choking (see page 135). Call for medical assistance.

Now your baby is one!

Your baby's first birthday marks a watershed for her and for you. You have had her for a whole year now, and she is so much a part of the family that you can't imagine life without her.

During this exciting and challenging first year she has changed from being a tiny newborn, dependent on you for her every need, to an energetic, enquiring child, who may already be toddling a few steps, or is on the threshold of walking alone. Having a baby has changed you too. As a parent you probably view the world differently from before. You now have a very real reason to think about the future and the kind of place the world will be when your baby grows up.

Although your baby is becoming independent, in many ways she is still just a baby. She continues to need the love, support and sympathy with which you have guided her through her first year. She will never again develop so rapidly, but there are many more new things for her to learn. She will continue to make good progress if, as you have done this year, you allow her to develop at her own pace.

She is beginning to have a mind of her own, but she has not yet learnt how to cope with the anger and frustration she feels when she discovers she is unable to do something she wants to do. Although you shouldn't let her have her own way all the time, getting angry with her constantly will not help either. You need a great deal of patience and humour to see you through the typical temper tantrums of the next year or so.

As you look back over the past year you will remember times when it all seemed too much. But you'll also remember the unrivalled sense of joy and achievement you felt as your baby smiled at you for the first time, waved goodbye to you as you went out, or greeted you for the first time by name. Over the next few years your baby will continue to grow in independence. It is your job to help her achieve this, always being guided by her needs at each stage. During the past year you have learnt to be sensitive to your baby's cues. As her unique personality continues to emerge you will get to know her better. Now as you look back, it is also a time to look forward too. The whole of that enchanted time, childhood, lies before you both – enjoy it!

INDEX

USEFUL ADDRESSES

National Childbirth Trust, Alexandra House, Oldham Terrace, Acton, London W3 6NH. Tel: 01-992 8637

Meet-a-Mum Association (MAMA), 5 Westbury Gardens, Luton, Beds LU2 7DW. Tel: 0582 422253

Pre-school Playgroups Association, 61 King's Cross Road, London WC1X 9LL. Tel: 01-833 0991

Association for Post-natal Illness, 7 Gowan Avenue, London SW6. Tel: 01-731 4867

Crysis, BCM Cry-sis, London WC1N 3XX. Tel: 01-404 5011

La Leche League (breast-feeding help and advice), 27 Old Gloucester Street, London WC1V 3XX. Tel: 01-242 1278

Association of Breast-feeding Mothers, 18 Lucas Court, Winchfield Road, London SE26 5TJ. Tel: 01-778 4769

Breast-feeding Promotion Group (same as National Childbirth Trust)

Mother & Baby

MAGAZINE

your pregnancy and childcare expert

With a baby on the way, it is important to keep track of the latest developments on all aspects of motherhood, from conception through to the early years with your new baby.

Mother & Baby magazine is Britain's best monthly guide, packed with exclusive reports and lively features for you and your growing family.

Regular sections on pregnancy and birth, your baby and toddler, family relationships and health and medicine offer factual information and expert advice which will continue to support you throughout the coming months and years . . . Plus a special colour section on the lighter side of motherhood, with fashion tips for you and your child, things to make and do, and lots of free gifts and special offers in every issue.

So make sure you don't miss a single issue of **Mother & Baby**. Have the next 12 issues delivered straight to your door, postage free, for only £12.00 – plus a full money-back guarantee if you decide to cancel at any time!

Simply call our *Subscription Hotline* direct on 0235 865656 with details of your Access or Visa card, and we'll take care of the rest. Or, if you prefer, complete the coupon below and post the whole page to:

Mother & Baby, FREEPOST, PO Box 35, Abingdon, Oxon OX14 3BR.

Yes, please send me the next 12 issues of **Mother & Baby** magazine, for only £12.00, postage free. I understand I can cancel at any time and receive a full refund.

Name

Address

Postcode   Tel. no.

A8490

I enclose cheque/PO for £ made payable to **Mother & Baby**

Please debit £ to my Access/Visa card, no.

Signature

Expiry date